SIMPLE EXERCISES TO STIMULATE THE VAGUS NERVE

Lars Lienhard
Ulla Schmid-Fetzer
with Dr. Eric Cobb

This English language edition published in 2021 by
Lotus Publishing
Apple Tree Cottage, Inlands Road, Nutbourne, Chichester, PO18 8RJ

Important note
The content of this book has been researched and carefully verified to the best knowledge and belief of the authors and publisher, against sources they consider to be trustworthy. Nevertheless, this book is not intended as a substitute for individual fitness, nutritional and medical advice. If you wish to seek medical advice, please consult a qualified physician. The publisher and the authors shall not be liable for any negative effects directly or indirectly associated with the information given in this book.

Editor: Markus Born
Cover design: Marc-Torben Fischer, Munich
Cover images: Shutterstock/Sebastian Kaulitzki
Models: Lisa Pfasch, Marina Schulik von Elace Sportmodels, www.elace-sportmodels.com
Layout: Medlar Publishing Solutions Pvt Ltd, India
Typesetting: Katja Muggli, www.katjamuggli.de
Printing: Replika Press, India

British Library of Cataloguing in Publication Data
A CIP record for this book is available from the British Library
ISBN 978 1 913088 17 0

SIMPLE EXERCISES TO STIMULATE THE VAGUS NERVE

An Illustrated Guide to Help Beat Stress,
Depression, Anxiety, Pain and Digestive Problems

Lars Lienhard
Ulla Schmid-Fetzer
with Dr. Eric Cobb

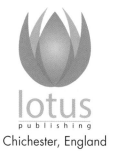

lotus
publishing
Chichester, England

Contents

Introduction

Many health problems, such as digestive disorders, chronic pain, blood pressure, breathing difficulties or circulatory problems, as well as emotional manifestations like anxiety or depressive moods, often result from our inability to process and cope with the ever-increasing stimuli and demands that the modern world throws at us. The efficacy with which our system – as in, our body and our central nervous system – navigates and responds to these growing requirements is often a crucial factor in our physical, mental and emotional health. These days, our nervous system is constantly in action mode, which often comes at the expense of regeneration and recovery. However, there are things we can do ourselves to improve the situation. If you're holding this book in your hands, it's probably because you want to change something about your life and your health. Perhaps you've noticed that things haven't been going as planned for a while now, or perhaps this feeling has come on all of a sudden. Or maybe you have the sense that there are things that should feel different. Perhaps you simply want to do something positive and invest in your long-term health, in which case, that's wonderful! Whether you want to reduce the symptoms of stress, change your lifestyle or just generally improve your fitness, this book will show you new ways to achieve these goals for yourself.

For some time now, the vagus nerve and its therapeutic effects have been the focus of significant interest, especially in terms of the development of different (self-)treatment options. A close look at the functions and roles of this important nerve shows that its stimulation can have a direct influence on relaxation, recovery and regeneration. When it comes to regulating the nervous system, there is no doubt that activating the vagus nerve is one of the most important tools we can use. However, the vagus nerve works neither independently nor autonomously. Even more important is the network in which it functions. One part of the brain that is especially significant in this respect is known as the insular cortex. You will see this term come up time and time again throughout this book. The insular cortex is the brain area where signals from within our bodies are coordinated with information drawn from our surroundings. The latest neuroscientific findings show that our awareness of our body's internal processes, also known as interoception, forms the basis for our resilience and our ability to combat stress.

Improving the way we process information from within the body and from our surroundings is the basis for a healthier nervous system and therefore holds the key to treating a variety of complaints and symptoms of stress.

With this book, we will be with you every step of the way on your personal journey to better health and wellbeing. In the first chapter, we will provide a basic introduction to the roles of the brain and the nervous system and how they work. The focus will be on the systems that have the capacity to relieve symptoms of stress and bring a greater sense of calm and inner balance. In the following chapters, we will equip you with a variety of exercises and training programmes that you can do at home to support your own health and healing. Whether your aim is to alleviate chronic pain, depressive moods or digestive problems, or you simply want to feel more calm and relaxed, you will soon notice an improvement in your symptoms – but only if you persevere with the exercises.

In fact, that is probably the most important message for you to take away with you: no one has ever been healed by reading alone. So, keep an open mind, keep practising and your hard work will pay off!

Lars Lienhard
Ulla Schmid-Fetzer
Dr Eric Cobb

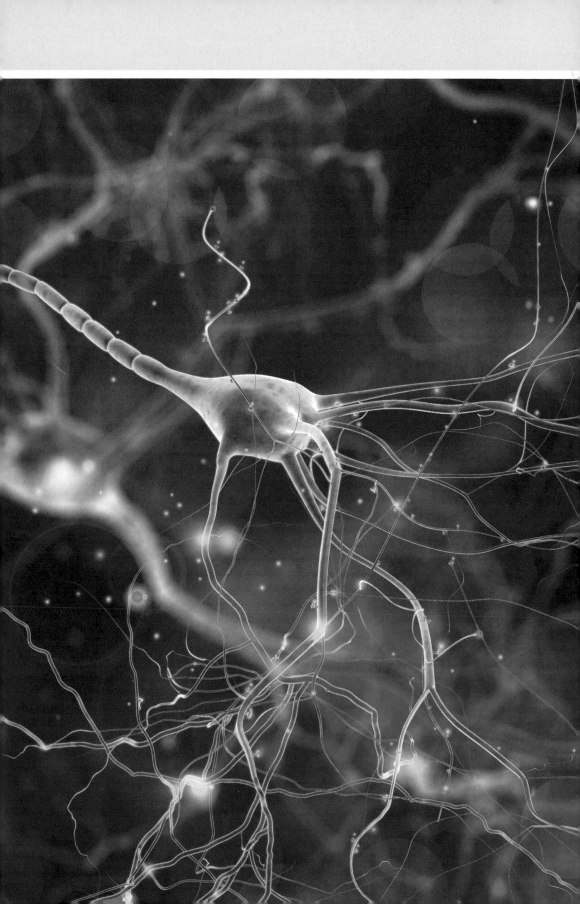

1

The significance of training the vagus nerve and interoception

The role of the brain and nervous system

If you want to take back control of your physical, mental and emotional health, it's crucial that you pay attention to the intricate workings of your brain and nervous system. The brain and the nervous system control and regulate all the processes in your body. You can think of your brain as the CEO of your body. Focusing on the neural connections and the laws of neural networking will not only help you to understand and categorise your symptoms and problems, but will also give you new ways to actively improve your health. We're talking here about the brain and the neural pathways, rather than any mental or psychological factors that are often associated with this topic. This book is more interested in the processes of receiving and processing information – in other words, the 'software running in the background'.

The fundamental aim of the brain and nervous system is to protect the body from danger and to keep it fit and healthy. In simple terms, this involves three significant steps:

- Step 1 – Input: Via the different sensory organs, the nervous system receives information from the surrounding environment, the body's movements and all its internal processes, such as organ activity and breathing, and transmits this information to the brain.
- Step 2 – Interpretation: These pieces of information are then integrated, analysed and compared with one another.
- Step 3 – Output: The information evaluated is then used to create a plan of action, which is sent to the different parts of the body so it can be implemented.

To avoid any misunderstandings, let's take a deeper look at the term 'action' as how the output commands are actualised in the body. The action we're talking about does not just refer to activities that are performed on a conscious level, which is how the word 'action' is understood in general usage. Rather, the actions referred to in this context are unconscious processes instigated within the body, such as those that regulate blood pressure, adapt the respiratory rate, coordinate muscle tension when moving, or control the formation of emotions and thoughts.

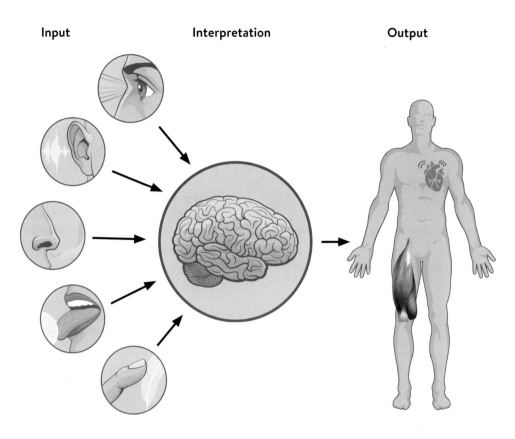

Input　　　　　**Interpretation**　　　　　**Output**

How the brain and central nervous system work: they receive sensory input, which they then process and integrate in order to initiate the next course of action.

Your physical wellbeing, fitness, health and behaviour are largely determined by the quality of the information your brain and central nervous system receive, transmit and process. The range of information received by your brain passes through a sort of 'danger filter', which is made up of different parts of the old brain. These parts, which developed early in our evolutionary history, use their integration and analysis functions to 'check' whether what you are about to do seems safe. If the brain isn't sure what is going to happen, it will interpret the situation as unsafe. It's important for you to understand that these processes are unconscious and happen as quick as a flash. In other words, your brain evaluates what's currently happening in your body and your surroundings in a fraction

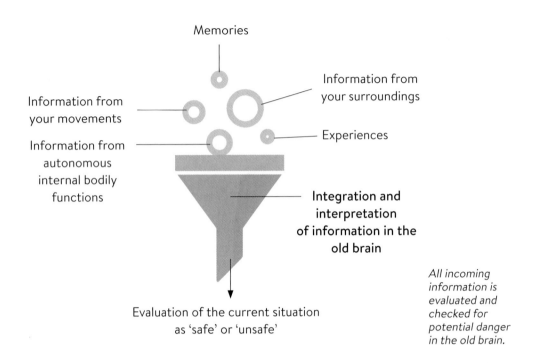

Memories

Information from your movements

Information from your surroundings

Information from autonomous internal bodily functions

Experiences

Integration and interpretation of information in the old brain

Evaluation of the current situation as 'safe' or 'unsafe'

All incoming information is evaluated and checked for potential danger in the old brain.

of a second, and constantly refreshes this information. To get some idea of the scope and complexity of this 'danger analysis', you need to know that the information your brain has to evaluate and assess is coming from every single part of your body. For example, at any given moment your brain is analysing information from all your blood vessels, your lungs, your joints, tendons and muscles in both halves of your body, your vestibular system and from both eyes and ears. Have you ever wondered about the quality of the information inside you? How would you evaluate the information from your own body?

All this information is analysed each millisecond and is used to determine, to a large extent, the perceived threat or danger to your brain. This is not just about recognising genuine danger, but also judging the predictability of the situation, which is based on the quality and quantity – or lack thereof – of all the signals coming in at any one time. Insufficient information, including that from within your own body, is interpreted by the brain as unpredictable and often as threatening. If that is the case, one specific part of the nervous system is activated more powerfully: the sympathetic nervous system. This system is responsible for making us more vigilant and alert in dangerous, stressful or demanding situations.

The counterpart to that is the parasympathetic nervous system, which soothes us and supports recovery. Although both systems are supposed to function simultaneously and in constant interplay with each other, this can quickly lead to an imbalance, at the expense of the parasympathetic system. In order for these two essential elements of the nervous system to resume equilibrium, a sort of 'mediator' is required. This is where the insular cortex or *cortex insularis* comes in. It is only in recent times that the insular cortex has started to receive more and more attention from the scientific community, who have realised what a significant role it plays in our sensory world and interoceptive awareness. It is examined in more detail from page 20 onwards. One of its many functions is to regulate the relationship between the parasympathetic and the sympathetic nervous systems.

In order to improve our health and wellbeing, we have to ensure that the information we receive from our surroundings, our own movements and from within our own bodies is clear and of good quality. This gives our brains a distinct sense of predictability and therefore safety. This allows the brain to regulate all processes at the optimum level, providing the basis for health, wellbeing and fitness.

Of course, the reception and processing of information about the current situation is not the only decisive factor here. Another important element is the correlation and comparison of this information with previous experiences, events or fears, which enables us to better judge the current situation. If the rules that govern the nervous system are not taken into account, it can be very difficult to establish the causes of problems which may have been affecting you for some time. Your brain's primary concern is to clearly predict a situation, for which it requires any information that can shed light on the current situation.

The quality of this information and its processing forms the basis for the next steps and the actions taken. This means that, if the incoming information is inadequate in terms of its quality or quantity, or if the activity level of the parts of the brain whose role it is to process this information is so high that they are unable to tell the brain that what's happening is clear, safe and predictable, then the actions and physical processes will be adapted to reflect exactly this message. If this diminished 'protective mode' is maintained over a longer period of time, your body's processes and basic functioning will gradually adapt to these new conditions, which are far from optimal. This ultimately manifests in a permanently diminished state of physical, mental and emotional health and well-being. Possible manifestations of this include: reduced mobility and strength, poor motor control, pain, dizziness, undesirable situation-specific emotional states, digestive or weight problems, as well as more complex phenomena such as symptoms of stress or anxiety, poor body image, difficulties controlling impulses, excessive muscle tension, or constant hypervigilance or combativeness leading to sleep disturbances.

In light of this, all physical processes and all symptoms can ultimately be tracked back to the brain and the central nervous system inadequately receiving, transmitting, processing or integrating sensory information.

How the nervous system is structured

Let's now take a closer look at the human nervous system. As complex and unique as this might seem at first glance, its basic structure is actually quite well organised and is the same for everybody. Almost every process in the human body is controlled by the nervous system. Its roles can be roughly divided into two main areas:

- Physical movements and/or the facilitation thereof.
- Maintenance of vital functions. These functions are for the most part autonomously regulated, i.e. they are involuntary.

The nervous system consists of one central system comprising the brain and spinal cord, as well as a peripheral system comprising all the other parts. The peripheral system is further divided into the somatic nervous system (which controls movement) and the autonomic nervous system, which is responsible for regulating autonomous functions such as digestion, breathing or regulating your blood pressure and heart rate.

This book pays special attention to the autonomic nervous system, specifically how it interacts with the central nervous system and the brain through its processing and control functions.

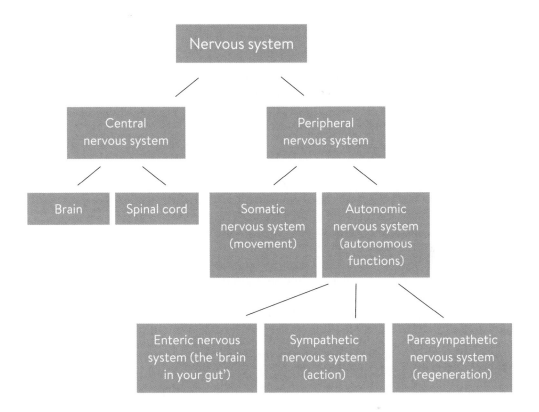

The nervous system is divided into two main parts – central and peripheral – which, in turn, are further divided into the somatic and the autonomic nervous systems.

The autonomic nervous system: the sympathetic and parasympathetic nervous systems

The three components of the autonomic nervous system are the sympathetic nervous system, the parasympathetic nervous system and the enteric nervous system (ENS). The enteric nervous system is also known as the 'second brain' or the 'brain in your gut' and is an almost entirely self-contained structure. Despite being very important to our health, the enteric nervous system is not an essential part of the topics covered in this book. Our key focus is on the sympathetic and parasympathetic nervous systems, due to their functions and roles within the body. The sympathetic and parasympathetic nervous systems work together to control the autonomous functions of the body, and therefore to maintain the internal balance between performance and recovery. The sympathetic nervous

Increasing resilience with a strong insular cortex

It's hard to define exactly what 'stress' is, and the same goes for its impact on the body. We often think of stress as something external – things we need to do or expectations we have to meet. This is why people often say they are 'under a lot of stress', for example. That said, this phrase also incorporates the feeling of being stressed, which in turn describes our physical and emotional reactions to these external (and internal) conditions.

But why do some people respond to difficult situations with (chronic) stress, while others seem to effortlessly recover from them? The ability to cope with stress factors and react well to experiences that derail us is known as 'resilience'. This is a subject that has received a lot of interest over the past few years, especially as it becomes increasingly clear how difficult it is to create a world without problems or unforeseen events. And here comes the fascinating part: it turns out that there is a correlation between resilience and the ability to efficiently interpret information from inside the body. This means that those with a greater capacity for accurately perceiving and interpreting their bodies and their internal conditions also have more resilience and are better able to deal with external stress factors – a highly desirable asset.

As you will see, the ability to perceive the body's internal processes and to establish their significance is controlled by the insular cortex. So, if this is working efficiently and is sufficiently active, you will be equipped to deal with the challenges – both big and small – that life throws at you.

system deals with action and response, while the parasympathetic nervous system is responsible for rest and recovery. So, when you need to be active, the sympathetic nervous takes over and ensures that all the systems required for productiveness are activated. Then, when you come to rest and relax, the parasympathetic system is activated and initiates the processes required for regeneration.

At a time when the outside world and the daily rhythm of most people's lives are becoming increasingly faster and more hectic, there are fewer opportunities for genuine rest, and even our free time is often spent carrying out highly stimulating activities. All of this places a great deal of pressure on the nervous system and can lead to disproportionate activation of the sympathetic nervous system. Without sufficient rest and regeneration, the brain gradually loses its ability to adequately regulate and compensate for these stress factors. The various possible symptoms of stress can affect us on many levels, from digestive disorders to increased blood pressure, unwanted weight gain, anxiety and exhaustion. From a neurocentric perspective, symptoms of stress are the end result of several processes that take place in the brain and nervous system.

The most important question here is this: How can we encourage a healthy relationship between our sympathetic and parasympathetic nervous systems and increase our resilience? After all, this is the only way to establish a healthy relationship between tension and relaxation and improve our health, wellbeing and fitness.

The vagus nerve – the main transmitter of information from inside the body

In order to balance out the activity of the sympathetic nervous system, it is important to do things that have a positive impact on the parasympathetic nervous system and regulate the relationship between the sympathetic and the parasympathetic nervous systems. In this respect, the vagus nerve – as the largest and most important nerve in the parasympathetic system and, as we will see later, one of the main sources of information for the insular cortex – is of particular importance. If we want to use the vagus nerve in a targeted way, we need to understand how this nerve fits into the overall structure of the nervous system and what role it plays. Let's start by considering the following questions: What does the vagus nerve do? Why is it so important?

The primary function of the vagus nerve is to absorb information from the body and send it to the brain. The vagus nerve also transports information from the brain to the organs, but this is more of a peripheral function. Only about 20 per cent of its fibres are what we would call efferent (i.e. descending) fibres. They send information and instructions from the brain to the body in order to initiate and regulate the autonomous processes, such as the abovementioned organ activity. This efferent pathway is also how anti-inflammatory signals are sent into the body, for example. Among other things, this is a significant factor in rheumatism, allergies and any symptoms relating to inflammation of the internal organs, and is therefore of great importance to our health and general wellbeing.

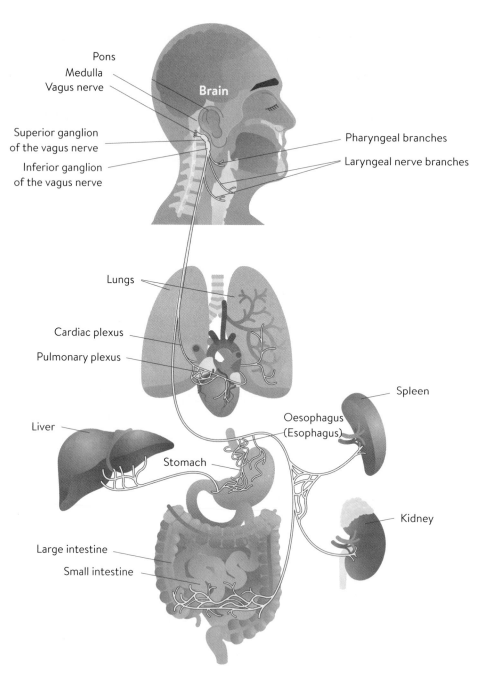

Pons
Medulla
Vagus nerve
Brain

Superior ganglion
of the vagus nerve
Inferior ganglion
of the vagus nerve

Pharyngeal branches
Laryngeal nerve branches

Lungs

Cardiac plexus
Pulmonary plexus

Spleen

Liver

Oesophagus
(Esophagus)

Stomach

Kidney

Large intestine
Small intestine

The vagus nerve mainly runs through the thorax and abdomen and innervates several internal organs.

If you look at the course of the vagus nerve, you will notice that it spans the abdomen, heart, lungs, large parts of the mouth and throat, scalp and ears. It innervates these parts of the body and is therefore responsible for transmitting information between these areas and the brain. This is extremely unusual for one single nerve – in fact, the vagus nerve is the only nerve that runs through the body both as a peripheral nerve and as a cranial nerve, and also innervates areas of the head. The nerve has a wide-ranging course, which branches off in lots of different directions, hence its name 'vagus', which comes from the Latin *vagari*, meaning 'to roam' or 'to wander'. The vagus nerve is therefore known as 'the wandering nerve', because it has many tiny offshoots that meander through large parts of the body.

Interoception – how we perceive what's happening inside our bodies

Irrespective of its size and ramifications, the type of information received and transmitted by this nerve is extremely important. The significance of the information that comes from within the body cannot be overstated. For one thing, this nerve delivers information about the respiratory system – one of, if not the most vital process in your body. It also delivers information about changes in blood gases, heart rate and blood pressure, as well as the activities and condition of the organs. For example, mechanoreceptors – which register the level of gastric distension in your stomach – feed back information about how full you are and therefore regulate your hunger levels. Chemoreceptors deliver information about chemical processes such as fluctuations in the pH value and oxygen levels in your blood, while thermoreceptors monitor temperatures and temperature changes in different parts of your body.

All this information from the vagus nerve gives the brain an idea of what exactly is happening in the unconscious processes that take place around your body. The brain's awareness of this information is called 'interoception', from the Latin *inter*, meaning 'inside' and *recipere*, meaning 'to receive'. Interoception is a model which is used to describe the way our brains perceive and regulate what's happening in our bodies. Along with the vagus nerve, there are several other components involved in this system. Interception incorporates all the systems that receive and transmit information, all the parts of the brain that process and integrate this information, as well as all the systems involved in the evaluation of this information. The interoceptive system is therefore not only responsible for receiving and processing, but is also heavily involved in initiating regulatory processes based on the information received. Normally, the function of the system is to maintain the internal state of the body or to adapt it for changing requirements, such as during exertion, while practising sports or exercising, or even in changing weather conditions. However, if our interoceptive awareness is not clear and accurate, the brain is unable to adequately predict our internal conditions, resulting in our responses – i.e. the output of the brain – being inadequate or disproportionate to the situation.

The concept of interoception or 'interoceptive awareness', in which the vagus nerve plays such a key role, forms the basis for the training programme described in this book. The main aim of these exercises is to increase our interoceptive accuracy by improving the way we receive and process information, and therefore how accurately our brain is able to predict the present situation. As one of the most important transmitters of information within the interoceptive system, stimulating the vagus nerve is an essential part of improving our interoceptive input. We will pay particularly close attention to this in Chapter 4 'Breathing and the pelvic floor' and Chapter 5 'Tongue and throat'. We will also be laying the foundations for better interoceptive awareness by carrying out the exercises in Chapter 3 'Mastering the basics' and Chapter 6 'Enhancing interoceptive awareness – touch, hearing and sight'.

The insular cortex – the control centre for interoception

Let's now look at the phenomenon of interoception in a little more depth. We have already established that the vagus nerve plays a mediating role in the transmission of vital information from around the body. You can probably imagine how immensely important the parts of the brain are that process and integrate this information. Based on the information they receive, these parts of the brain enable us to regulate the autonomous functions of the body as efficiently as possible. When you look at these regions of the brain, there is one that particularly stands out: the insular cortex. The insular cortex is where the majority of the information

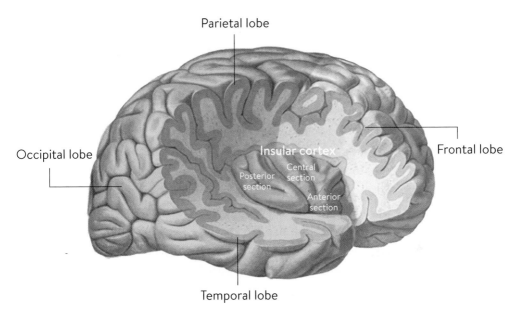

Parietal lobe

Occipital lobe

Insular cortex

Central
Posterior   section
section

Anterior
section

Frontal lobe

Temporal lobe

The insular cortex is a small part of the brain located deep inside the cortex and is responsible for interoception.

received by the vagus nerve gets sent. It is a cerebellar structure located deep inside the cortex, between the frontal, parietal and temporal lobes.

It's only in recent years that the insular cortex has started to receive more and more attention from the scientific community. And yet, we already know that it is involved in a wide range of important functions. As a significant integrative centre within the brain, the insular cortex helps to regulate the autonomous, unconscious functions of the autonomic nervous system. It thereby exerts a considerable influence on the interplay between the sympathetic and the par-asympathetic nervous systems. It analyses information from within the body (interoceptive signals), compares it with other sensory information, integrates it and assigns it an emotion, making it – to all intents and purposes – the body's interoceptive 'headquarters'.

The brain and the nervous system depend, to a large extent, on knowing how these vital processes work and are assessed. If this information is insufficient, for whatever reason, this can render us unable to regulate our internal processes efficiently. This causes a range of unwanted 'side effects', which may affect our breathing, organ activity, blood pressure or digestion, for example.

In order to ensure the optimum interoceptive awareness, and thus to coordinate the key aspects of our health as efficiently as possible, our insular cortex has to integrate all this information perfectly, while also comparing and relating it to our memories, experiences and fears. Interoception – or interoceptive awareness – can therefore be described as the subjective perception and mapping of the inner state of the body, which is based on the information received by the brain and nervous system. This not only includes information relating specifically to our physical bodies, but also any psychological, mental and emotional factors, too. At first glance, you could be forgiven for assuming this process is so incredibly complex that there is very little possibility of influencing it. However, this is simply not the case. That's because, as described, these integration processes take place in the insular cortex and, like any other part of the brain, the insular cortex is constantly adapting to changing conditions – which means it is able to be changed and trained!

In the next section, we will take a closer look at the structure and the various functions of the insular cortex and show you how you can improve its activity level with targeted exercises.

Structure and functions of the insular cortex

The insular cortex is roughly divided into three areas: the posterior (rear) section, the central section and the anterior (front) section. Looking more closely at the roles of each section – the posterior section of the insular cortex processes the raw sensory data from inside the body as well as from our movements, feelings and surroundings. The central section integrates this information, compares it with the data from all the other senses and analyses it. In the anterior section, this data is then compared with previous events, memories and experiences. This results in a cognitive assessment and consciously perceived emotions.

According to most definitions, the anterior section is also part of the cerebrum, i.e. the higher parts of the brain that are linked to awareness and cognition.

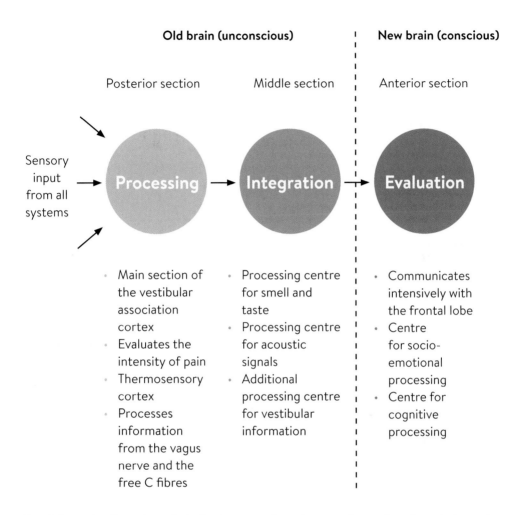

Most information flows through the insular cortex from the posterior section, through the centre towards the anterior section.

Most of the information that passes through the insular cortex moves from the back to the front. To improve the general activity level, our main focus is on addressing the two rear sections. This heightens activity in the whole area and leads to a general improvement in all functions of the insular cortex.

The insular cortex also contains other subsystems or 'centres' whose job it is to evaluate and integrate specific information. These centres are located in the different sections of the insular cortex. Targeted stimulation of these centres is a very effective way to tap into the various sections of the insular cortex and therefore to improve their key functions. Let's look at a few examples: One important centre is what's known as the vestibular association cortex, located in the **posterior section** of the insular cortex. This compares vestibular information with all our other sensory impressions. Training the vestibular system (Chapter 3, page 64 onwards) is therefore essential when it comes to the general training and honing of our interoceptive awareness, as well as to the targeted stimulation of the posterior section of our insular cortex.

The centre for information relating to smell and taste is located in the **middle section** of the insular cortex. This processes and evaluates the intensity of smells and tastes and compares these impressions, asking itself: 'How does that make me feel?'. In terms of your training, this means that specific smell and taste exercises can be used to stimulate the central section of the insular cortex, thereby improving all associated functions. This can be particularly effective for people who have difficulty losing weight, as this is where the emotional components (special preferences, aversion, disgust) of taste are processed, among other things. The primary function of the central section, however, is to integrate all the sensory information, which means that – by tapping into this 'smell centre' – you can improve the general integration processes of the insular cortex.

The **anterior section** of the insular cortex is where the socio-emotional centre is located, which has several functions, including determining the way in which we engage with and deal with the feelings of others. This centre is involved in emotional disorders such as social anxiety, panic attacks and depressive episodes. The anterior section of the insular cortex also has direct communication links to higher parts of the cortex, and to the frontal lobe in particular.

You can make excellent use of all these specific areas and connections to regulate and stimulate the various sections of your insular cortex and their roles and functions. As you will see, it is possible to target specific areas and to improve their functionality.

The key functions of the insular cortex

Due to its range of functions, connections and interactions, the insular cortex plays a fundamental role in many different processes:

- Awareness of internal conditions within the body (interoception)
- Control and regulation of the intestinal muscles (digestion)
- Evaluation of the intensity of pain and patterns of chronic pain
- Perception and regulation of heat and cold (thermosensory cortex)
- Regulation of breathing and control of blood pressure and pulse
- Adaptation of autonomous functions during exercise and stress
- Integration of vestibular information
- Hand-eye coordination and motor learning
- Swallowing and articulation
- Regulation of the autonomous nervous system and the interaction between sympathetic and parasympathetic tone
- Regulation of the immune system
- Body awareness and ownership – the sense of being in control of your own body
- Processing of the feeling of disgust towards odours and images
- Awareness and identification of fundamental emotional responses (fear, anger, irritation, joy, sadness)
- Guiding and maintaining attention

If there is a dysfunction in this extremely important part of the brain, it can cause difficulties when it comes to performing these functions, as well as an imbalance in the regulation of the sympathetic and parasympathetic nervous systems. This in turn can lead to a variety of symptoms. The imbalance in the autonomic nervous system can cause stress symptoms to accumulate and can also impair the regulation of autonomous functions. One outcome of this is that it affects digestion and organ activity, increasing the likelihood of problems such as digestive problems, sensitive stomach or acid reflux. Another frequent outcome is that the autonomous functions have difficulty adapting to changing conditions and levels of exertion, such as shortness of breath when climbing stairs or engaging in exercise and sports, etc. It is also common for difficulties in motor learning, problems with coordination, and issues with posture and stability to appear when the activity level of the insular cortex is impaired. Furthermore, dysfunctions in this vital part of the brain are also known to cause disorders of the immune system such as rheumatic diseases, allergies and autoimmune diseases.

As mentioned previously, one of the key functions of the insular cortex is to assign emotions to information about physical aspects of the body, which means that any dysfunctions in the insular cortex can result in a whole range of problems when it comes to regulating emotions. This can range from inappropriate laughing or crying and difficulties interpreting feelings and emotions, to more serious problems such as anxiety disorders and depression. In particular, if information from inside the body can be perceived but cannot be interpreted accurately, the higher parts of the brain (the cortex) turn to memories and their meaning to try to establish what the physical sensation could mean. This can result in thirst signals being misinterpreted as hunger, for example. This 'top-down regulation' of the insular cortex often goes hand-in-hand with an overactive anterior section, especially in the case of anxiety disorders and depression. Those affected then tend to focus excessively on and over-interpret all the sensations within the body. Further information can be found in Chapter 7 from page 247 onwards.

Overview of the potential effects of a dysfunction of the insular cortex and interoception

- Irritable bowel syndrome, bloating and acid reflux
- Eating disorders
- Excessive anxiety, anxiety disorders and depressive moods
- Difficulties correctly categorising the intensity of pain – this can make everything seem incredibly painful, for example
- Difficulties interpreting or understanding feelings and emotions
- Inappropriate laughing or crying
- Difficulties processing traumatic events
- Lack of body ownership – the sense of not being at home in your own body
- Motor disorders and problems with motor learning
- Difficulties identifying acoustic signals
- Problems adapting the cardiovascular system and breathing to exercise and stress

- Dizziness or balance problems
- Travel sickness
- Heightened awareness of your own heartbeat
- Difficulty swallowing
- Chronic immune disorders such as allergies
- Problems with sensory integration
- ADHD and other attention disorders
- Pelvic floor problems

If you look at the wide range of pathologies that can develop if your interoceptive awareness is not functioning as well as it ought to, it's no wonder that it is often so difficult to improve individual symptoms. Attempting to treat individual symptoms in isolation is usually far less effective than considering the symptoms in their wider context and incorporating into your training the functions and functioning of the neural systems that operate in the background. The practical part of this book is therefore devoted to improving these neural processes and functional connections – in other words, improving the way we record and interpret information for a better output. We will be focusing mainly on the insular cortex, which is responsible – among other things – for establishing the right balance between the sympathetic and the parasympathetic nervous systems, which is ultimately the basis for a healthy, happy and less stressful life! However, before you get started with the training, we would like to give you a brief overview of what this book has in store for you and how to get the best out of it.

How to use this book

We hope that the introduction to the neural networks at play in the brain and nervous system, as well as interoceptive awareness and its importance for health, wellbeing and fitness, has shown that you have the power to take these things into your own hands. Now that you have an understanding of the neural structures working in the background, what they do and how they are connected to one another, you can focus on improving your input and interpretation, and therefore make a positive impact on your interoceptive awareness and autonomous regulatory processes.

Chapter by chapter, we will guide you through the various aspects of improving your interoceptive awareness. For each subject area, we will give you a series of simple and effective exercises that you can carry out almost anywhere and at any time, with very little effort. In the next chapter 'Assessments – quick tests for lasting success' – we will first show you ways of evaluating how each of the exercises is affecting your own nervous system. This way, you can keep checking which exercises are working well for you and which ones you might want to put on the back burner. These assessments are essential for getting the best out of the training and making it work for you. In each chapter, you will find a list that you can use to work out how the tests for each of the exercises went.

In the first part of the exercise section of the book – from Chapter 3 (page 53) onwards – you will find the basic framework in which the entire interoceptive process takes place. Here, we will give you a set of exercises specifically designed to improve this framework, creating the best possible foundation for your interoceptive awareness training. Chapters 4 and 5 on pages 117 to 211 are designed to train individual aspects of interoceptive awareness, focusing specifically on breathing and the pelvic floor as well as giving sensory stimulus to the tongue and throat. As you will see, stimulating the vagus nerve plays a particularly important role here. Other important aspects that influence our interoceptive awareness and the activity levels of the insular cortex and parasympathetic nervous system include pressure massage, sensations of warmth and cold, localising and differentiating acoustic signals and relaxing the eyes. This wide range of aspects will be covered in Chapter 6, from page 213 onwards. In Chapter 7 (page 247 onwards), we will focus on targeting the anterior section of the insular cortex through body awareness and mindfulness exercises.

Finally, in Chapter 8, starting on page 263, we will teach you how to combine and plan the exercises you have learned in order to improve specific problems or symptoms. Here you will find training plans and exercise combinations for improving digestive problems, chronic pain, pelvic floor problems, emotional regulation and general wellbeing, as well as for reducing stress and increasing fitness levels.

In each of the chapters, we will show you which area of the insular cortex is addressed through that particular training process and which pathologies can be alleviated by the special exercises. This will enable you to take back control of your own health!

Exercise according to your own needs

Because interoception is such a complex integration process, we recommend certain exercises at the end of each chapter. These allow you to either train individual systems such as your respiratory system or your tongue, or to integrate individual exercises into your personal interoceptive awareness training. Because the nervous system is so individual, we can't tell you in advance which aspect will be most important for you. However, this book will provide you with a wide variety of exercises to choose from, so that you have the best possible options for improving your health. However, don't let this variety throw you off. Any exercise that gives positive assessment results can be built into your training and will have a positive impact. The one crucial thing is that, whichever exercises you choose, you need to spend a total of at least 20 to 30 minutes per day on your training if you want to make changes that are sustainable and effective. You can focus on one element or put together your own training plan made up of two or three elements – whatever works for you!

Train regularly to stay healthy as you get older

By using the exercises in this book, you can take your health back into your own hands and take vital steps towards having more zest for life and improved wellbeing and fitness. You can use your newly acquired neuroscientific knowledge in specific ways in order to improve particular aspects of your life – more quickly and more efficiently. One of the most important lessons is the fact that the brain and nervous system have incredible neuroplasticity and therefore have the ability to adapt to new conditions. This means that your brain has the capacity to change and to improve – even into old age and in spite of any difficulties you may be experiencing. What an amazing thing for you to focus on in your training! As a general rule, training for 20 to 30 minutes each day over a course of six to eight weeks is enough to effect the desired neural changes. Of course, you are welcome to practise for longer. So let's get started and look forward to seeing the results!

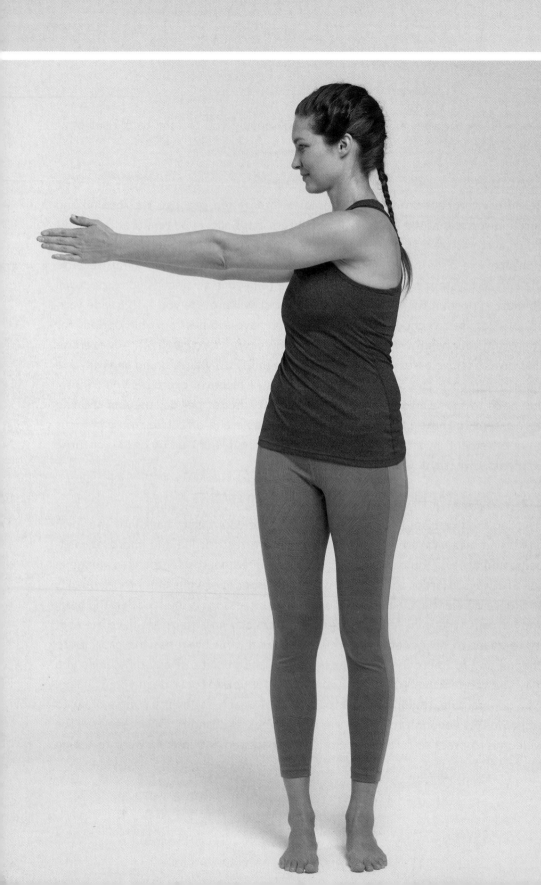

2

Assessments – quick tests for lasting success

Test the effectiveness of your training

In order to achieve the best possible results from your training, you need to check how effective each exercise is for you. Our nervous systems are as individual as our fingerprints, and every one of us will respond differently to the training. You can only create the best possible training schedule for you if you know how your own nervous system responds to the exercises. People often claim that certain exercises always have a positive effect on them, but – from a neuroscientific perspective – this is not necessarily the case. If you don't test it, all you have is guesswork. The nervous system is the fastest and most adaptable system in the body and responds immediately to any new information it receives and processes.

As we have already seen in Chapter 1, the brain receives information from the body and the environment (input), evaluates it and integrates it. Based on the evaluation of this information, a plan is created, which is then sent to the organs, such as the muscles, lungs and heart, where the plan is implemented. That's the output. And you can check the quality of this output using these short, uncomplicated tests or assessments. Working out how your system responds to the different exercises is crucial for the progress of your training. Does the output improve? Does it remain unchanged or possibly even get worse? Depending on the results of the assessment, the effect of each exercise can be categorised and used to create the most effective training plan for you.

Feedback from a training partner

At first, it can sometimes be difficult to notice changes in yourself. Everything often feels the same and you may not be able to tell right away if and how the training is affecting you. If you are unsure about your test results, you are welcome to carry out the assessments together with a training partner. They can then document your flexibility from an external perspective, for example, or time you while you're holding your breath or performing long muscle contractions. Furthermore, a training partner can sometimes be a better judge of whether you appear calm and relaxed during the exercise and the assessment, or whether you tense up, impacting the quality of the movement. Having a training partner assess your body language can be another way of helping you get the best out of the exercises. The better your interoceptive awareness becomes, the more reliably you will be able to evaluate your own assessments. Take your time and don't be afraid to get support in the early stages.

Without testing the effects of each exercise, you can only make assumptions and won't know for sure whether or not the exercises and routines you perform will actually improve your own nervous system. We therefore encourage you, as you work through this book chapter by chapter, to test each exercise for yourself and to record the results of the assessments in the tables at the end of each chapter. This will make it easier for you to put together your individual exercise plan. Instructions for the exercise plans can be found at the end of each chapter and in Chapter 8 (page 263 onwards), in which we suggest a variety of special exercise combinations. These are designed to help you reduce your symptoms effectively and sustainably.

How to use the assessments

The process is really simple. First, carry out one of the assessments described below, such as the 'forward bend' flexibility test (page 37). Then, do your exercise, such as bag breathing (page 160), and then repeat the assessment. If your performance in the assessment has improved – so, in this example, if you have greater flexibility after the exercise – then you can assume that the exercise carried out had a positive effect on your nervous system. You can mark this in the corresponding table. If you didn't notice any change, or only noticed a moderately positive change in the assessment results after the exercise, then you can assume it had a neutral effect. You should write this down in the table too. As a basic rule, you should feel free to incorporate into your training plan any exercises that had a positive or neutral effect.

However, if your performance in the assessment is worse after carrying out the exercise, then you can assume that your nervous system was unable to clearly perceive the exercise and therefore deemed it a threat. We would therefore say that the exercise had a negative effect. There's no need to worry about this – after all, that's precisely what we're trying to find out. It's all about assessing the effects of the exercises on your nervous system, without bias or judgement. So, if the information that is sent to your brain while you're performing an exercise is classified by your brain as not being sufficiently predictable, this will always be directly reflected in the output. In this case, we simply need to adapt the intensity of the exercise so that it has a positive effect for you. Make a note of this in the table and, if possible variations are given, test these out. If you still don't achieve a positive or neutral result, put the exercise to one side for now and use those that do have a positive effect instead. The exercises can be divided into three categories according to the results of the assessments:

- Positive: These exercises have the greatest positive impact on your nervous system and on improving your interoceptive awareness. After performing these exercises, you see a significant improvement in your assessment results.
- Neutral/moderately positive: These exercises have a neutral to moderately positive effect and can be integrated into your training right away. In order to achieve even more positive effects, you can adjust their intensity or combine them with other exercises.
- Save for later: These exercises are currently having a negative impact on your system. If you don't achieve any positive effects despite having tried different variations, then this exercise should be tested again at a later date.

Testing is important, but shouldn't cause stress

If you find the idea of 'being tested' difficult and it gives you added stress, then simply start with the exercises that you enjoy. You can return to the assessments later, once your stress level has returned to normal.

It's all in the method

In the beginning, certain exercises may still cause you 'stress', even though you are already on the right track with your training. There are various things you can do to help deal with these exercises.

- Reduce the intensity of the stimulus a little, i.e. the speed or the amount of movement, for example during vestibular training.
- Reduce the resistance you are working against when training your respiratory muscles, for example.

- Adjust the duration of the exercise in order to achieve a positive effect. In other words, do the exercise for less time and take a few breaks in between.
- Increase the duration of the exercise if you feel that it will have more of an effect.
- Change the order of the exercises within your training plan and then repeat the assessment.
- Perform the exercises a little more intensively and for longer than specified.

In each chapter, we will advise you on ways in which you can modify the exercises. You may find that you have to postpone certain exercises or elements that cause you more stress for the time being and test them again later. In this case, simply carry on with the exercises to which you respond positively. This is perfectly fine and will not reduce the effects of your training. In practice, it is often the case that, after a short time, exercises that initially caused you stress end up having positive results.

A little exercise can make a big impact

Don't underestimate the effect of the exercises! Despite appearing simple or even inconsequential at first glance, certain exercises may have more intense effects than you first thought.

Assessment 1 – Mobility

One quick and easy assessment is checking your mobility. The exercises introduced in this book as a way of improving your interoceptive awareness, as well as the parts of the brain stimulated by these exercises, have a significant impact on your 'stretch tolerance'. This term refers to the amount of stretch or traction on the tissue that your brain and nervous system will tolerate. Your stretch tolerance largely determines how flexible you are. This means that, if you improve the function of the parts of the brain that evaluate and assess your interoceptive awareness, this will almost always result in increased mobility. On the following pages, we will show you three different mobility tests that you can use to assess the effectiveness of the exercises and your overall training. Choose a test that makes you feel safest and most comfortable. For example, if you are having major problems with your balance, a forward bend is probably not the right exercise for you. In that case, you may wish to start with the shoulder mobility assessment to test the effects of your training.

❯ Forward bend

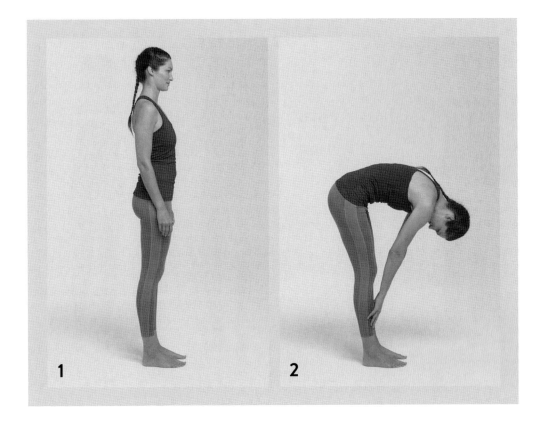

1

2

1. Stand up straight with your feet hip-width apart. Lengthen your spine but keep it nice and relaxed. Allow your breath to flow smoothly and evenly, with a relaxed gaze straight ahead. Let your arms hang loosely by your sides.
2. From this position, bend forward as far as you can and – without bending your knees – see how far down you can bend, trying to touch the floor, your toes or the bottom of your calves with your fingers. Feel the tension in the back of your body and make a note of how far you can bend down. Repeat the test two or three times to get a basic idea of how flexible you are. The amount of tension in your back and your range of motion will be used as a benchmark for the retest.

› Body rotation

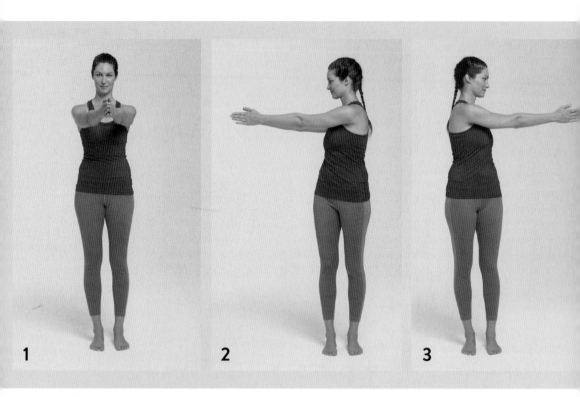

1

2

3

1. Stand up straight with your feet hip-width apart. Lengthen your spine but keep it nice and relaxed. Allow your breath to flow smoothly and evenly, with a relaxed gaze straight ahead. From this position, raise your arms up in front of you to shoulder height – without bending your elbows – and place your palms together.
2. Now rotate to the right two or three times, as far as you can go.
3. Then rotate two or three times to the left. Make sure that your feet stay pointing forwards and do not rotate with you. If one side is a little less flexible than the other, this will make a very good reference point for the assessment. Make a note of your range of motion as well as the level of tension you feel when rotating your body. This information can be used as a benchmark for the retest.

❭ Shoulder mobility

1. Stand up straight with your feet hip-width apart. Lengthen your spine but keep it nice and relaxed. Allow your breath to flow smoothly and evenly, with a relaxed gaze straight ahead. Bend your right elbow 90 degrees and lift your arm sideways to shoulder height.

2. From this position, rotate your arm outward two or three times as far as it will go by turning your arm backwards and upwards. Come back to the starting position.

3. Then rotate your arm inward two or three times by turning your arm backwards and downwards. Come back to the starting position. Then switch sides and do the same exercise but with your left shoulder. If one side is a little less flexible than the other, this will make a very good reference point for the assessment. Make a note of your range of motion on each side, as well as the level of tension you feel. This information can be used as a benchmark for the retest.

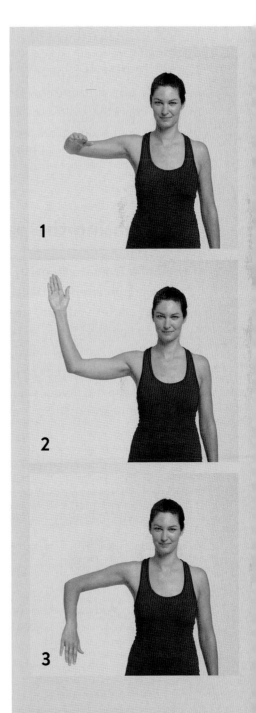

Assessment 2 – Pain level

In addition to mobility tests, classifying your own pain level is another suitable assessment you can use to check for any improvement in your interoceptive awareness. Pain perception is closely related to the functionality of the insular cortex. As you already know from the first chapter (page 25), the insular cortex plays an important role in evaluating how intensely we feel pain. If you feel less pain after your training, this would indicate that the function of the insular cortex has improved as a result of the exercises.

❭ Evaluating the pain level

If you suffer from pain regularly or even experience chronic pain, it makes sense to use your perceived pain level as an assessment. Considering the type of movement that causes you pain, start to perform this movement in a controlled and relaxed manner and focus on the pain. How severe does the pain feel on a scale of 1 to 10? 1 is a very, very mild pain, while 10 is as severe as it gets. Make a note of where on the scale your pain level is. You will use this number as a comparison for the assessment. If your pain level is lower down the scale after performing an exercise, you can classify the exercise as 'positive'. If you also feel pain while at

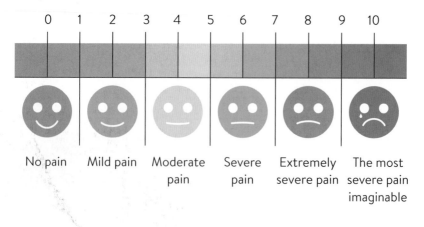

How severe is your pain? Use this scale to help identify your pain level.

rest, rate this pain according to the scale too, as we just described. There is no need to perform any additional movements that may induce even more pain.

Test your pain level regularly

Of course, there are also pain symptoms and pain conditions for which improving interoceptive awareness results in no immediate change, or very little change. You should test your subjective pain level at regular intervals in order to assess and classify the long-term progress of your training. As a general rule, you will find that your mobility and range of motion will improve first, and then you will see a reduction in pain levels.

Assessment 3 – Air hunger

The amount of time you can hold your breath for without experiencing severe air hunger gives a good indication of how well your brain is able to assess the physical condition of your body. Holding your breath and the biochemical changes it triggers in the body require the insular cortex to correctly classify and regulate the change in oxygen and carbon dioxide levels in the blood. If you cannot stand the feeling of being short of breath or if your brain reports 'danger' very early on, this would indicate that your brain has a limited ability to correctly assess information from inside your body. For this reason, timing how long you can hold your breath for without feeling severely out of breath is an ideal way to assess your interoceptive awareness. If the amount of time you can hold your breath for calmly and easily increases after carrying out an exercise, then the exercise has a positive result.

Listen to your body!

Some people can find holding their breath extremely uncomfortable or scary. Please only use this assessment if you feel safe doing so, and do not overdo it.

Generally speaking, we have enough oxygen in our bodies to hold our breath for more than 30 seconds without feeling an urgent impulse to breathe in. In practice, however, those of us with dysfunctional interoceptive awareness have a strong urge to inhale much earlier than others, and some people are unable to control or suppress this impulse. It often feels like you need to breathe in after only a few seconds. The purpose of the assessment is to observe how the brain responds. All the exercises in this book can improve your ability to hold your breath and to endure the feeling of breathlessness. If this assessment is still too uncomfortable for you at the beginning, use the other assessments first and come back to this one in a few weeks' time.

❯ Hold your breath

Equipment: Stopwatch

Stand up straight with your feet hip-width apart. Lengthen your spine but keep it nice and relaxed. Look straight ahead with a relaxed gaze. Close your mouth, and cover your nose if necessary. Start the stopwatch. Hold your breath for as long

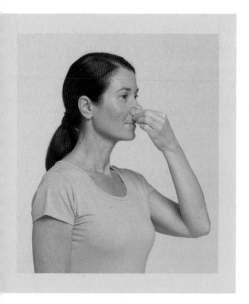

as you can tolerate and control the feeling of breathlessness. Please do not force yourself to hold your breath for longer than is comfortable. After all, it is an assessment and not a competition! Make a note of the time from which you find breathing so uncomfortable that you have an urgent impulse to breathe in or to swallow. This time will be used as a comparison for the retest. Please make sure the same conditions are in place each time you carry out the 'hold your breath' assessment. This will give you the most accurate indication of how effective the exercises have been. It's up to you whether to inhale or exhale before holding your breath. Do whichever you find most comfortable.

Note: If you are particularly worked up or you have been physically exerting your-self, this will affect your capacity to hold your breath and to endure or control the urge to inhale. This, in turn, will affect the results of the assessment.

Assessment 4 – Muscular contractions

Another way of assessing how well your interoceptive awareness is improving is to test how long you can hold a muscle contraction. This requires good regula-tion of autonomous functions. For example, prolonged muscular tension leads to changes in blood pressure, blood flow and intramuscular pressure, which then need to be adjusted adequately. And these autonomous functions are regulated by the insular cortex. Our capacity to sustain prolonged muscular tension is there-fore an indicator of the function and activity level of the insular cortex.

In the following exercises, we will create muscular tension through a series of sim-ple holding exercises on the right and left sides of the body. Your task is to hold this tension for as long as possible. If the assessment shows that one side of the body has less stamina, this would indicate that the central nervous system does not have the capacity to sufficiently regulate autonomous functions during mus-cle contraction. If you find it easier to generate and hold muscular tension after performing the recommended exercises, this would suggest that your brain's capacity to control these autonomous functions has improved.

Moderate exhaustion is plenty

The muscle contraction assessment can be quite exhausting. It's therefore unnecessary to continue until you reach maximum muscle exhaustion. You will usually notice very quickly the point at which it becomes difficult to maintain the muscle contraction, or when the muscle tension on one side of the body significantly decreases.

❯ Holding muscle tension

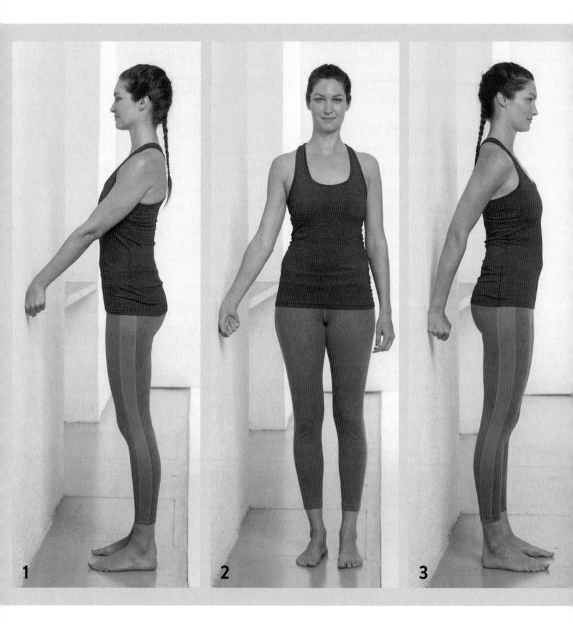

1. Stand with your feet hip and shoulder-distance apart, facing a wall or door frame at a distance of around 50 to 60 cm. Lengthen your spine but keep it nice and relaxed. Allow your breath to flow smoothly and evenly, with a relaxed gaze straight ahead. Make a loose fist with your right hand and bend your elbow slightly. Press your fist against the wall, with your thumb and index finger making contact with the surface. Start by applying light pressure against the wall and then gradually increase it. Continue to build up the muscle tension for the next 5 to 10 seconds, at which point you should be pushing against the wall with as much strength as you can muster. Now continue to push against the wall with maximum force for as long as you can. Count in seconds how long you can hold this pose. Make sure to keep the rest of your body as stable and relaxed as possible. The force should only be coming from your arm.

2. Change position and press your arm sideways against the wall. Make sure that you start by building up the tension slowly, as you did before, and then hold the maximum tension for as long as possible.

3. Finally, turn so that you're standing with your back to the wall and press your right arm backwards against the wall, making contact with the wall with the outside edge of your hand and your little finger. Again, build the tension slowly and then hold the maximum force for as long as possible. Then switch sides and repeat steps 1 to 3 but with your left arm.

Note: Take care to always stand in the same position and the same distance away from the wall. Most people find that one side is much weaker than the other. It's best to use your weaker side for the assessment.

Assessment 5 – Balance

Another assessment you can do is to test your balance. The ability to maintain your balance is closely connected to the function of the insular cortex and your interoceptive awareness. The insular cortex contains what's known as the vestibular association cortex (pages 23–24). This is where information to do with our balance is processed, integrated and compared with other sensory information. The insular cortex also communicates with the central section of the cerebellum – the vermis. The vermis is heavily involved in core coordination and stability. If we can improve how vestibular information is processed and integrated, as well as making the vermis more active by increasing activity in the insular cortex, then this usually results in better balance and a more stable, secure standing position.

For the assessment, have your feet close enough together that it's difficult to maintain your balance. There are two options described below – the narrow stance and the tandem stance. If your exercise routine is working, you will find that you feel more stable, secure and in control when you repeat the balance tests, and that you can maintain your balance for longer.

› Narrow stance

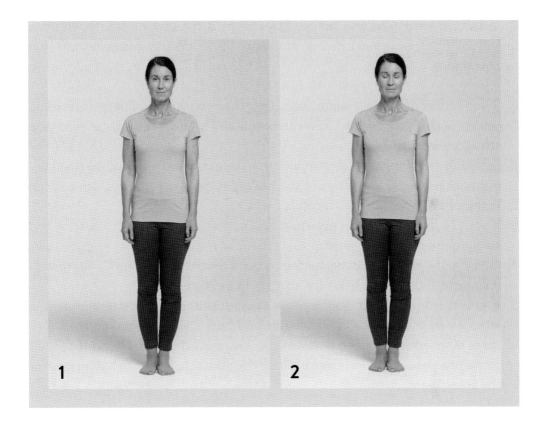

1. Stand with your feet hip-width apart. Lengthen your spine but keep it nice and relaxed. Allow your breath to flow smoothly and evenly, keeping a relaxed gaze straight ahead. From this position, close the distance between your feet to form a narrow stance. See how well you can balance for 15 to 20 seconds.
2. If you can, try closing your eyes to make the test even more challenging. Pay attention to how the stance and your balance feel. Are you able to maintain a stable and relaxed posture for the whole time? Or do you notice that you gradually start to sway and lose your balance? Make a note of how stable this stance feels for you and use this information as a benchmark to compare against later assessments.

〉 Tandem stance

An advanced version of the balance assessment is the tandem stance. Use this one if you find you haven't had or no longer have difficulty balancing with the narrow stance.

1. Stand with your feet hip-width apart. Lengthen your spine but keep it nice and relaxed. Allow your breath to flow smoothly and evenly, keeping a relaxed gaze straight ahead.
2. From this position, place your right foot in front of your left foot, so that your right heel is touching the tips of your left toes. See how well you can balance in this position for 15 to 20 seconds.
3. If you can, try closing your eyes to make the test a little more challenging and to get more conclusive results.
4. Open your eyes and switch your feet around so that you left foot is in front of your right. Hold this position for another 15 to 20 seconds.
5. If possible, try to close your eyes in this position too. Pay attention to the intensity of the balance requirements and how stable the stance feels. Are there differences between the two foot positions? If you find it more difficult to maintain your balance in one position over the other, use the harder one for the assessment.

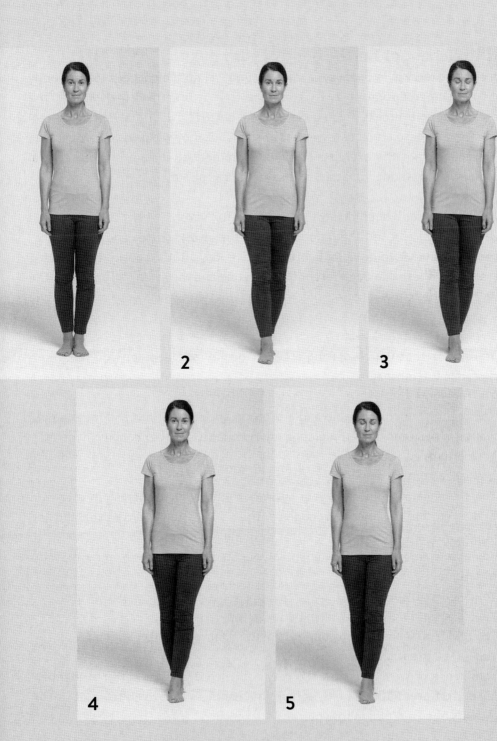

2

3

4

5

Positive changes for the good of your health

After each exercise, in one way or another you will notice changes to your body and to your perception of it. Try to notice if your breathing feels lighter and deeper after an exercise, if you generally feel better (in your body) or if you feel less stressed. These aren't assessments as such, but they will give you a clear idea of whether or not the exercise is having an immediate impact on your central nervous system – and ultimately, that's what it's all about.

If you have already been doing the exercises for several weeks or months and have gradually improved the functionality of the insular cortex and your intero-ceptive awareness, you will undoubtedly notice lots of other positive changes in yourself too. These can be different for everyone and they won't all appear at the same time. The following effects indicate a few ways in which your body and the way you feel may change:

- You notice that you're getting a better quality of sleep and you feel more rested in the mornings.
- You feel more motivated to get moving or do sports.
- You feel less uncomfortable and anxious in social situations and meetings as well as in busy and over-stimulating environments such as shopping centres.
- Your breathing feels easier, both while at rest and under exertion or during physical activity.
- You see an improvement in your awareness of what's happening in your own body. You find it easier to recognise when you're tense or relaxed and the intensity of any muscle soreness, for example.
- You notice an overall improvement in your stamina and have fewer symptoms of fatigue.
- You feel less bloated.
- You notice a reduction in inflammation.
- You feel less discomfort in your gastrointestinal region after eating.
- You have a greater sense of balance.
- Your sense of smell changes. You may notice that you get better at identify-ing and differentiating smells, or that you react less sensitively towards smells, if that's been a problem for you.

- You notice an improvement in your ability to swallow. You may find swallowing tablets and capsules less difficult, or eating and drinking may feel easier and more natural.
- You may well notice an improvement in your hearing.
- Your hunger and thirst levels return to normal. You have less of an urge to eat to make yourself feel 'good'.

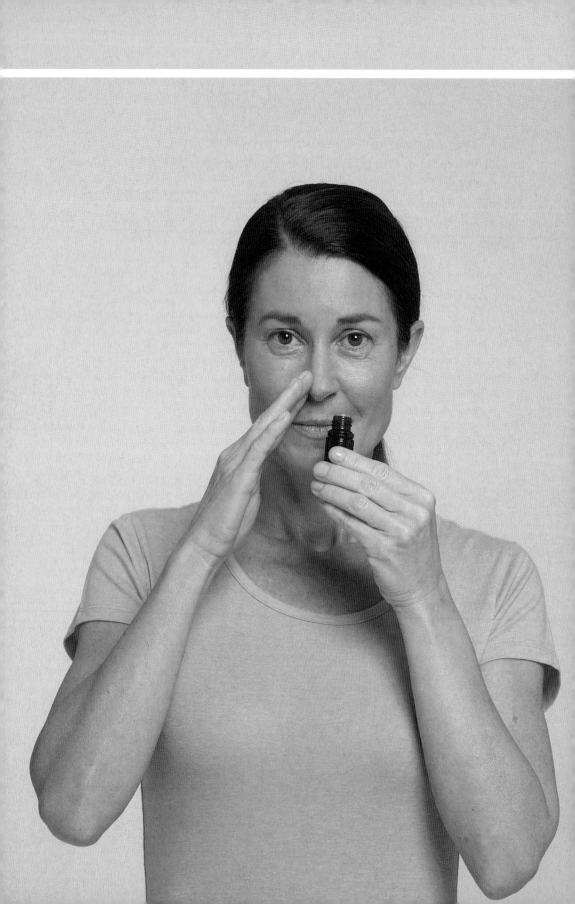

3

Laying the foundations for optimal vagus nerve training

The importance of preparing the vagus nerve and interoceptive awareness training

As you know from the first chapter, our interoceptive awareness is an incredibly complex and multi-faceted neural phenomenon. For this reason, it is particularly important for us to focus on the parameters within which the perception and regulation of information takes place. These parameters can be seen as all the elements of your brain and nervous system that, irrespective of what's actually happening inside the body, interact closely with the insular cortex and affect its functionality. These elements hold the key to increasing your interoceptive awareness, raising your fitness levels and improving your overall health.

This chapter is about building the proverbial 'framework' for your further training, to maximise the impact of your training and make sustainable improvements to your interoceptive accuracy. In Chapters 4 to 7, we will be showing you how to train individual components that each have a major impact on your health in and of themselves, helping to reduce stress, improve fitness and give you a greater sense of wellbeing. It is of course possible to train each element individually, but it is only by creating a strong foundation – i.e. by establishing the optimum parameters – that you can really make headway with your training.

We have designed this book to offer you a comprehensive and holistic perspective on this issue, focusing on the neural principles and relationships that govern your health and wellbeing. Our main focus will be on stimulating the frontal lobe, an area of the cortex that communicates intensively with the insular cortex, as well as improving the functionality of the vestibular system, which forms the basis of the entire nervous system. The vestibular system in particular is so crucial to the functions of the insular cortex and interoceptive awareness that we strongly recommend making this a focal point for your training. We will also be stimulating the central section of the insular cortex – which is also crucial to the integration of sensory data – with a series of exercises involving smell and taste. We will then focus on straightening and elongating the cervical spine and mobilising the vagus nerve, in order to improve the mechanical components involved in the transmission of information between body and brain. At the end of the chapter, you will find additional options for stimulating the supplementary motor areas (page 110). These make up an important section of the frontal lobe, which is heavily involved in the coordination and regulation of internal processes. As you work through this chapter, you will see that the better the parameters are, the more effectively you will be able to train the individual components of your interoceptive awareness. And the overall result? Better health, a greater sense of wellbeing, and improved fitness.

Upregulating the frontal lobe

If you look at how the insular cortex communicates with other parts of the brain, you will see that a significant quantity of information is exchanged between the frontal lobe and the insular cortex. One of the most important roles of the frontal lobe is to control or suppress unwanted impulses. The brain has to respond to incoming stimuli and give permission to the body to perform or prevent an action: a 'go signal' from the brain performs an action, while a 'no-go signal' stops it. Go and no-go signals are processed in specific areas of the frontal lobe. If the no-go signal is missing or arrives too late, the unsuppressed impulses trigger inappropriate and disproportionate reactions. This results in your brain using old solution strategies and behaviour patterns, which are often unable to adequately solve the situation. Whether you have difficulties turning down that delicious piece of cake, even when you're no longer hungry, or breaking a spiral of unhealthy thoughts – any form of behaviour change relies on the 'no-go signal' and needs it to be triggered quickly, before the brain just goes into autopilot and does what it usually does.

Exercises that strengthen and train the frontal lobe are particularly effective when it comes to improving your ability to respond adequately to impulses. The exercises in this chapter stimulate the relevant areas of the frontal lobe and allow you to process stimuli related to your interoceptive awareness, such as feelings of hunger or thirst, in a more differentiated, more appropriate and more effective way, giving you more control over your impulses.

❯ Saccades – quick horizontal eye movements

One simple and easy way to activate the frontal lobe and the posterior section of the insular cortex is to do horizontal eye movements called saccades. The initiation and neuronal organisation of this movement takes place in the frontal fields of the eye, which are part of the frontal lobe and are in close proximity to the area that is jointly responsible for our ability to inhibit impulses. Because they are often supplied by the same blood vessels, parts of the brain that are close to one another each have an impact on the other's activity levels. If you activate the frontal fields of the eye by jumping between different visual targets, you stimulate and increase the blood supply to the part of the frontal lobe that is responsible for suppressing impulses. Stopping the movement of the eye when it lands on the visual target is coordinated by the opposite cerebellum. This reports the precision of the eye movements directly to the frontal lobe, prompting it to optimise the movements if necessary. This communication forces the frontal lobe to work harder, meaning that it is activated both directly by triggering the eye movements and indirectly by stopping the eyes on the target. The posterior section of the insular cortex in particular is stimulated by the movement of the eyes. Increasing the activity level of the posterior section of the insular cortex helps you to reduce stress and regulate pain more effectively.

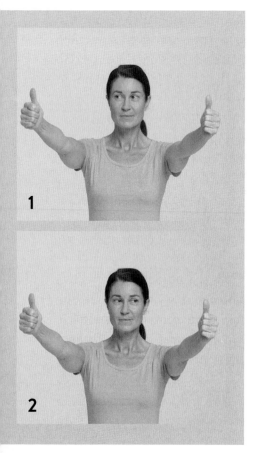

1

2

1. Stand up straight with your feet hip-width apart. Lengthen your spine but keep it nice and relaxed. Allow your breath to flow smoothly and evenly. Lift your arms up to eye height, without bending your elbows and with your thumbs pointing to the ceiling. Focus both eyes on your right thumb.
2. For a duration of 30 to 90 seconds, switch your focus to and fro between your right and left thumb. Make sure that your head stays still.

› Saccades with training cards

Equipment: Two saccade cards

To make the eye movement exercise more interesting and varied, you have the option of using special training cards called saccade cards. These force your eyes to switch between left and right, line by line, as you jump from one letter to the next. This variation of the eye exercise requires more concentration and more precise eye coordination in order to find the right letters on the right line each time you switch. This also increases activity in the frontal lobe.

N	Y
X	W
Y	T
W	M
S	P
M	M
P	S
O	W
L	D
K	E
U	D
I	F
O	G
P	T
Z	Y
K	J
B	L

1. Stand up straight with your feet hip-width apart. Lengthen your spine but keep it nice and relaxed. Allow your breath to flow smoothly and evenly. The training cards should be positioned in front of you at eye level, around 60 to 80 cm away from you.
2. Focus on the first letter on the left-hand training card.
3. For a duration of 30 to 90 seconds, switch your focus to and fro from the right to the left card and back, line by line, working through the block of letters from top to bottom. Make sure that your head stays still.

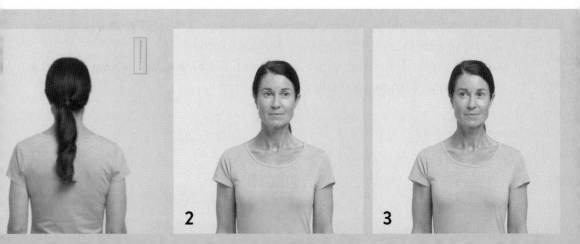

2   3

❯ Anti-saccades – a special type of eye movement

Probably the most effective eye exercises for activating the exact region of the frontal lobe that suppresses impulses are what we call anti-saccades. This exercise is about suppressing an impulse generated by a visual stimulus and instead performing the opposite action. As you have already seen, every time you are forced to suppress an impulse – i.e. control your response to a stimulus – your frontal lobe becomes more active. The visual system is designed in such a way that your eyes reflexively jump to an object as soon as you notice a conspicuous movement in your peripheral vision. This allows you to identify what the object is and whether or not it poses a threat. This exercise requires you to suppress your natural and deeply ingrained instinct to look at the visual stimulus. So, you receive a visual stimulus, suppress your natural response to it and instead move your focus away from the stimulus. This special type of eye movement intensely activates areas of the brain that are involved in impulse control. The exercise also requires a lot more focus and attention than the saccades and thus also activates the anterior section of your insular cortex. Anti-saccades are therefore a useful and effective means of activating this important part of the insular cortex, which has a positive impact on your emotional regulation. All you need for this fun and extremely effective exercise is a training partner.

1. Stand up straight with your feet hip-width apart. Lengthen your spine but keep it nice and relaxed. Allow your breath to flow smoothly and evenly. Have your training partner stand about a metre and a half away from you with their arms outstretched at eye height. First, rest your gaze on your partner's forehead or, depending on how tall they are, their chin.
2. Your training partner will now begin to make a rocking or waving motion with their index and middle fingers, which you should only notice in your peripheral vision, as your focus is still on their forehead or chin.
3. As soon as you notice the finger movement, switch your focus away from the moving fingers to your training partner's other hand.

4. From there, return your gaze to your partner's forehead or chin. Carry out this exercise for 60 to 90 seconds. It's important that your training partner keeps switching hands in an unpredictable sequence. This ensures you have to stay focused the whole time you're doing the eye exercise.

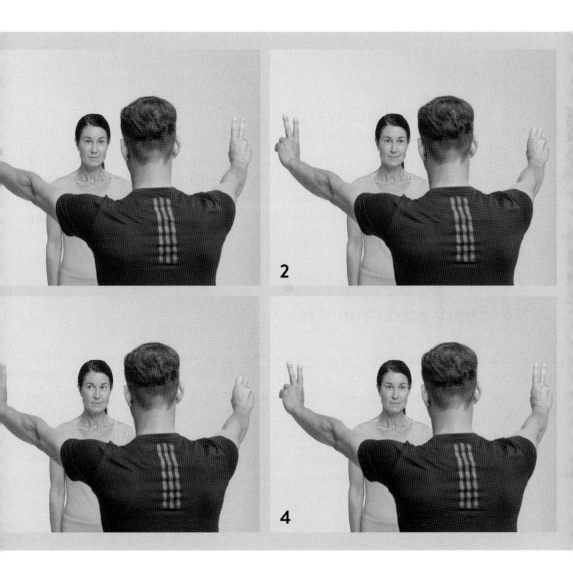

'Dual tasking' brain training exercises

Another fun way to activate the frontal lobe is to build counting exercises or specific brain-training exercises into your training or your daily routine. You can do these while carrying out other simple activities such as walking, jogging, climbing stairs, washing up or having a shower. By combining elements of movement and attention, these exercises stimulate the frontal lobe as well as the front and posterior sections of the insular cortex, and therefore improve your interoceptive awareness, as well as your general sense of wellbeing and your fitness levels.

❯ Counting backwards

While doing an activity of your choice, start to count backwards from 100 in increments of 7. So, you will be saying aloud, '100', '93', '86', and so on. It's important that you keep doing the activity as well as you can while counting. At first, you can try this exercise simply while walking, and then build up to more complex activities.

❯ Every other month

While doing an activity of your choice, start listing the months from January to December. The crucial trick is only to say every other month aloud. So, you would say 'January' aloud, then think 'February' in your head, then say 'March' and then think 'April', and so on. As with the counting exercise, it's important that you keep doing the activity as well as you can. As with the anti-saccades (pages 58–59), this exercise requires you to control and suppress your impulses – in this case, the impulse to say every month in the sequence aloud. In this way, the exercise directly addresses the important parts of the frontal lobe.

Brain-training apps and games

Other fun options for training the parts of the brain that are responsible for impulse control – and that communicate with the insular cortex – are apps and games specifically designed for this purpose. You can simply download them onto your smartphone, PC or tablet and use them whenever you have a bit of spare time, such as on the bus or train, during your coffee break, in the doctor's waiting room or at home. The games vary in terms of their structure and the way they test your reactions, so we have kept the following descriptions quite general. You will find more information in the game instructions provided by the manufacturers. We recommend the following apps for your training:

- **Stroop Test:** This game requires you to suppress your initial impulse to respond to the meaning of the word and instead respond to the colour in which the word appears. So, for example, you might see the word 'red', but written in green. Your task is to respond to the colour of the lettering (green) rather than the word itself (red).

- **Dual N-Back:** This game gives you a series of different prompts, which are always made up of two types of stimuli, e.g. one aural and one visual. Your task is to indicate when the current stimulus matches a stimulus that was displayed a certain number of steps before.

- **Go/No-go Games:** In these games, there are certain symbols or stimuli that you are supposed to react to, usually by pressing a key, and others that you're not supposed to react to. When playing these games, you should answer as quickly as possible, and pay close attention to ensure you react (or don't react) correctly too.

Categorising the exercises that activate the frontal lobe			
Exercise	Positive	Neutral/moderately positive	Save for later
Saccades – quick horizontal eye movements (page 56)			
Saccades with training cards (page 57)			
Anti-saccades – a special type of eye movement (pages 58–59)			

Categorising the exercises that activate the frontal lobe			
Exercise	Positive	Neutral/moderately positive	Save for later
'Dual tasking' brain training exercise (page 60)			
Counting backwards			
Every other month			
Brain-training apps and games (page 61)			
Stroop Test			
Dual N-Back			
Go/no-go games			

Training recommendations for activating the frontal lobe

Frontal lobe exercises can be used for four different purposes. One option would be to make these fundamental exercises the main focus of your training, in which case you would do just these exercises in isolation for 20 to 30 minutes each day for three to six weeks. Focusing solely on this area works particularly well for people who have difficulty responding to stimuli and suppressing impulses. This includes eating disorders, addictive tendencies and inappropriate emotional reactions such as anger, anxiety, depression, inappropriate laughter or frequently bursting into tears. You could also use frontal lobe stimulation to work towards creating a better foundation for the next stage of your training, either as part of your training plan or as preparation for other exercises. You could integrate the exercises into more advanced interoceptive training as a sort of 'warm-up'. If you're going to do this, pick one or two exercises that gave you particularly positive assessment results and build these into your training. Depending on their intensity, spend 2 to 5 minutes on them at the start of your routine. You can use the recommended games and apps (page 61) as a way of improving the general functionality of your frontal lobe. To do this, you should aim for a minimum daily training time of 10 minutes per day, divided into 2 to 3 minute frontal lobe training sessions that you would do four or five times throughout the day. This can be a fun thing to do during your coffee break, or just when you have a bit of free time.

Training recommendations for activating the frontal lobe		
Potential use	**Scope and application**	**Effect**
As the main element of the training	• Exercises with a positive or neutral/moderately positive assessment result • 20 to 30 minutes each day • Divided into 2 or 3 smaller sessions • Carried out over the course of 3 to 6 weeks	• Improves your ability to suppress your impulses and change your behaviour • Activates the anterior section of the insular cortex; anti-saccades (pages 58–59) and the Stroop Test (page 61) are particularly effective • Improves: • emotional regulation • anxiety • depressive moods • impulse control • symptoms of stress
As part of interoceptive awareness training	• 1 to 2 exercises with positive assessment results • 3 to 5 minutes each day	Saccades (page 56) and dual tasking (page 60) also activate the posterior section of the insular cortex and help to improve: • recovery and regeneration • symptoms of stress • chronic pain • interoceptive awareness • general wellbeing and fitness
As a warm-up for other training exercises	• 1 to 2 exercises with positive assessment results • 2 to 5 minutes • Immediately before carrying out further training	Improves the overall effectiveness of the training
As a leisure activity or during your break at work	• 2 to 3 minutes playing brain-training games or apps (page 61) • 4 to 5 times throughout the day	Improves impulse control

Optimising the vestibular system

The vestibular system has several important functions. It tells the brain where you are in relation to the space around you, which way's up and which way's down, and helps you to navigate your way through a space. The vestibular system measures acceleration and changes in position of the head and body, and sends this information to certain (key) areas of the brain. The brain uses this information to stabilise your movement and adjust your posture to the speed and direction of acceleration. The vestibular system also supports all the other important systems that help control your movement. It stabilises your vision and has a huge impact on your coordination and motor learning, as well as on the regulation of autonomous functions within the body.

One of the functions of the vestibular system is to help you counteract the force of gravity in order to keep your posture upright. The information it uses to counteract the effects of gravity is extremely important for the insular cortex and the regulation of autonomous processes. In response to this information, adjustments have to be made to your blood pressure, breathing, muscular activation, the regulation of your internal organs and much more – and this is where the insular cortex comes in. The extreme importance of the vestibular information is clearly evident when we look more closely at the anatomy of the insular cortex. In the posterior section, we find what's called the 'vestibular association cortex'. The term 'association cortex' simply refers to those areas of the cortex that integrate specific information and compare it with all other sensory information. In this case, the information is from your vestibular organs, and it is compared with information from elsewhere in your body as well as information taken from your surroundings.

However, vestibular information is not only processed in the posterior section of the insular cortex, which is primarily responsible for bodily functions, pain regulation and organ activity. The information also activates the central section of the insular cortex, which is connected to the hormonal system and integrates interoceptive signals. The vestibular system is therefore of significant interest when it comes to interoceptive awareness, improving digestion, reducing stress, evaluating pain levels adequately, as well as the regulation of our emotions and internal processes. It has a positive impact on almost all areas of our interoceptive awareness and therefore creates a framework for the regulation of autonomous processes.

The structure of the vestibular system

The vestibular organs, which measure acceleration, are located in the inner ear on both the left and right sides of your head. They each comprise three semicircular ducts (vestibular canals) and two otolith organs (the saccule and the utricle). The three semicircular ducts – horizontal, superior and posterior – are positioned next to one another at an angle of around 90 degrees. Their job is to measure angular acceleration, which is induced by rotation. In contrast, the otolith organs – the saccule and the utricle – measure linear acceleration. The saccule is responsible for upwards and downwards movements, while the utricle is responsible for forwards, backwards and sidewards movements.

However, the vestibular system does not only include the vestibular organs, but in fact all the components that are involved in the reception, transmission and processing of vestibular information. The vestibular system sets the frame of reference for all other systems and is one of the essential foundations of the nervous system. In the following section, we will start by demonstrating a few simple exercises that you can use to target the individual components of the vestibular organs. We will then move on to some slightly more complex and some combined vestibular exercises, which will challenge the vestibular system even more and will intensely activate the posterior sections of the insular cortex. This will help you to improve how information is received and processed by this vital system, and will create the best possible framework conditions for your interoceptive training.

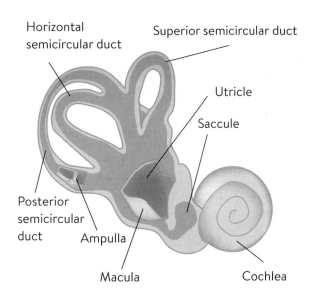

The vestibular organ located in the inner ear consists of three semicircular ducts, which measure the angular acceleration induced by rotation, as well as the macular organs (otolith organs) – the saccule and the utricle – which measure linear acceleration.

Seven basic vestibular training exercises

When beginning to train your vestibular system it is best to start with a few simple exercises that are particularly effective in achieving extensive, global activation of the vestibular system. The basic exercises we've chosen are 'no-no' and 'yes-yes' movements, as in shaking or nodding the head, and head tilts. With simple yet specific head movements, they hone in on the different vestibular canals in the inner ear (see figure on page 65). We will also show you a series of basic and more advanced variations that you can do to make the exercises more challenging.

❯ 'No-no' movements (horizontal)

Equipment: Two visual targets

The simplest exercise you can do to kick-start your balance training is what we call 'no-no' movements. When you look at the position and layout of the vestibular organs, it's clear to see that you can train the horizontal ducts on the right and left side of the vestibular system simply by rotating the head to the right and to the left. That's why 'no-no' movements are often used to target the horizontal ducts of the vestibular system. For the best results, lower your nose and chin slightly and keep them parallel to the ground while carrying out the movement. Try not to twist your neck or tilt your head to one side. Instead, keep it parallel to the ground at all times.

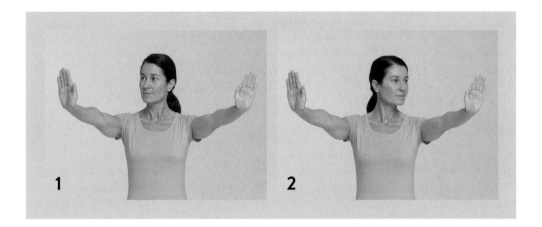

1. Stand with your feet hip-width apart. Lengthen your spine but keep it nice and relaxed. Allow your breath to flow smoothly and evenly. From this position, pick out two focal points at eye level to your left and right. You can also have your arms outstretched and use those as focal points for the exercise. Start by looking to the right, turning your head and gaze simultaneously.
2. Begin to accelerate your head from right to left with rapid, rhythmic 'no-no' movements. Continue this movement for 30 to 120 seconds. To begin with, pick a rhythm and speed that you find it easy to control, and increase this over time. The aim is to keep a steady rhythm, in which you can perform the entire cycle of movement from the right to the left and back again within one second.

❯ Variation 1: 'No-no' movements with eyes closed

Once you've mastered the basic version of the exercise, you can move on to doing the 'no-no' movements with your eyes closed. Taking away your visual orientation makes your brain even more reliant on receiving precise, clear vestibular information. It also increases your focus and, in turn, the efficiency of the exercise.

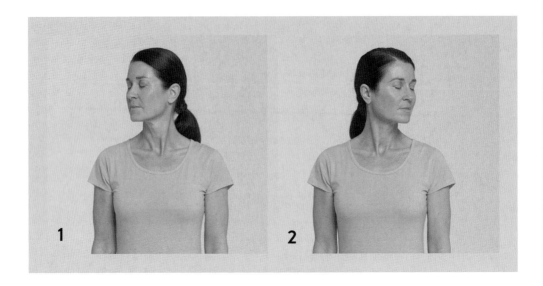

1. Stand with your feet hip-width apart. Lengthen your spine but keep it nice and relaxed. Allow your breath to flow smoothly and evenly. Close your eyes and turn your head to the right.
2. Begin to accelerate your head to the left and to the right with rapid, rhythmic 'no-no' movements. Continue this movement for 30 to 120 seconds. It's important to start out by picking a rhythm and speed that you feel comfortable with and find easy to control. Again, the aim is to keep a steady rhythm that allows you to perform the entire cycle of movement from the right to the left and back again within one second.

〉 Variation 2: 'No-no' movements with a clear visual target

Equipment: Visual target

For the next step up, carry out the 'no-no' movements while keeping your gaze fixed on a visual target. The ability to stabilise your eyes while your head is moving

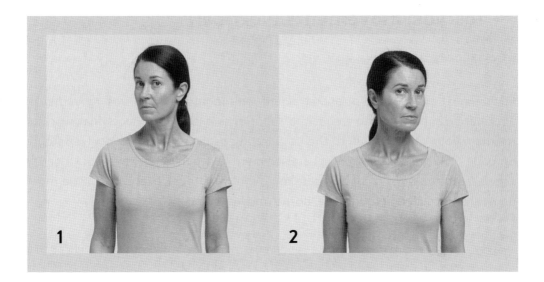

is, as mentioned previously, an extremely important aspect of balance training. Try to keep your visual focus as clear and stable as possible while you carry out this exercise, which is designed to train the horizontal ducts in your vestibular system.

1. Stand with your feet hip-width apart. Lengthen your spine but keep it nice and relaxed. Allow your breath to flow smoothly and evenly. Focus on a visual target positioned between 1 and 1.5 m in front of you, at eye level. Turn your head to the right, while keeping your eyes fixed on the target.
2. Begin to accelerate your head from right to left in a series of rapid, rhythmic 'no-no' movements, keeping your eyes on the target. Continue this movement for 30 to 120 seconds. It's important to start off at a speed that you feel completely comfortable with, and at which your focus on the visual target remains clear and unblurred at all times. Again, the aim is to keep a steady rhythm that allows you to perform the entire cycle of movement from the right to the left and back again within one second.

Note: Pick a visual target that's the right size to allow you to keep a focused view of it throughout the exercise.

❯ 'Yes-yes' movements (vertical)

Equipment: Two visual targets

For the next stage of the balance training, we recommend 'yes-yes' movements. These are a simple way to target the superior and posterior ducts that work to maintain your balance. Due to the layout and position of these ducts (see figure on page 65), the superior and posterior ducts are activated when your head is accelerated forwards or backwards. You might find these exercises a little more unusual and challenging than the 'no-no' movements.

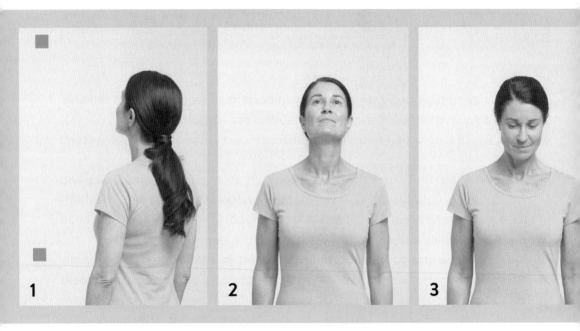

1. Stand with your feet hip-width apart. Lengthen your spine but keep it nice and relaxed. Allow your breath to flow smoothly and evenly. From this position, pick two targets – one above and one below your eye – that are pretty much aligned with one another.

2. First, lift your head and eyes up to focus on the upper target.
3. From here, begin accelerating your head and eyes down and up again between the two visual targets, with rapid, rhythmic 'yes-yes' movements. Continue this movement for 30 to 120 seconds. It's important to start out by picking a rhythm and speed that you feel comfortable with and find easy to control. The aim is to keep a steady rhythm, in which you can perform the entire cycle of movement from the upper to the lower target and back up again within one second.

Note: Try to keep your head straight during the whole exercise, and make sure it doesn't rotate or tilt to the side. To get a better sense of when your head is in the right place, you could work with a training partner. They can give you feedback until you have a better feel for your own head position.

❯ Variation 1: 'Yes-yes' movements with eyes closed

Once you've mastered the basic version of the exercise, you can move on to doing it with your eyes closed. As is the case with the 'no-no' movements, taking away your visual orientation makes your brain more reliant on clear, precise vestibular information, which makes the exercise more focused and more effective.

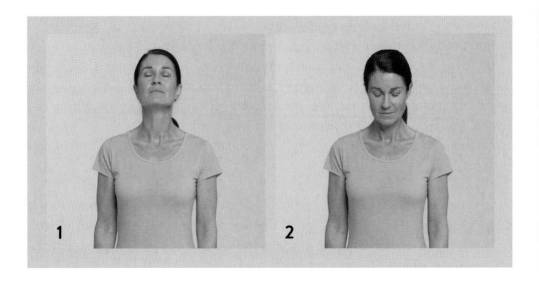

1. Stand with your feet hip-width apart. Lengthen your spine but keep it nice and relaxed. Allow your breath to flow smoothly and evenly. Close your eyes and start by lifting your head upwards.
2. Begin to accelerate your head downwards and back up again with rapid, rhythmic 'yes-yes' movements. Continue this movement for 30 to 120 seconds. It's important to start out by picking a rhythm and speed that you feel comfortable with and find easy to control. The aim is to keep a steady rhythm, in which you can perform the entire cycle of movement from the upper to the lower target and back up again within one second.

❯ Variation 2: 'Yes-yes' movements with a clear visual target

Equipment: Visual target

For the next step up, carry out the 'yes-yes' movements as described in Variation 1, but this time keep your eyes focused on a clear visual target – positioned directly in line with your eyes – for the duration of the exercise. The ability to stabilise your eyes while your head is moving is, as mentioned previously, an extremely important aspect of vestibular training. Try to keep your focus on the target as clear and stable as possible throughout.

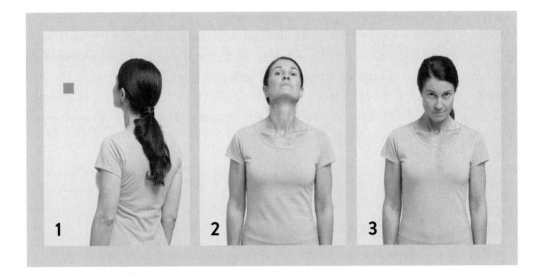

1. Stand with your feet hip-width apart. Lengthen your spine but keep it nice and relaxed. Allow your breath to flow smoothly and evenly. Focus on a visual target positioned between 1 and 1.5 m in front of you, at eye level.
2. First, point your head upwards while keeping your eyes on the target.
3. Now begin to accelerate your head downwards and back up again in a series of rapid, rhythmic 'yes-yes' movements, keeping your eyes on the visual target the whole time. Continue this movement for 30 to 120 seconds. It's important to start off at a rhythm and speed that you feel completely comfortable with, and at which your focus on the visual target remains clear and unblurred at all times. The aim is to keep a steady rhythm, in which you can perform the entire cycle of movement from the upper to the lower target and back up again within one second.

Note: Pick a visual target that's the right size to allow you to keep a focused view of it throughout the exercise.

❯ Lateral head tilts

Alongside the 'no-no' and 'yes-yes' movements, there is another simple and effective exercise that you can use to activate both the superior and anterior vestibular ducts as well as parts of the otolith system (see figure on page 65). This exercise involves tilting the head to the right and left in order to stimulate the vestibular system. Lateral head tilts are a little harder than the previous exercises because they require more coordination and more efficient interaction between the different components of your vestibular system. You should therefore only attempt this exercise once you have successfully pre-activated the brain with a series of 'yes-yes' and 'no-no' movements.

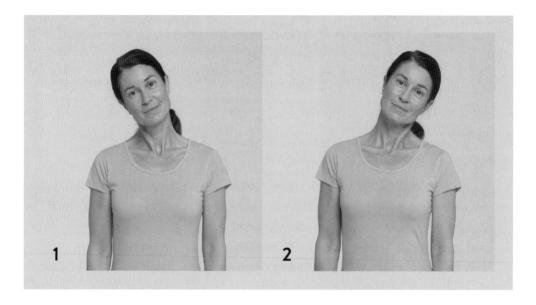

1. Stand with your feet hip-width apart. Lengthen your spine but keep it nice and relaxed. Allow your breath to flow smoothly and evenly. Tuck your chin slightly while lengthening your neck, lowering your nose by 2 or 3 cm. Then tilt your head to the right.
2. Start to tilt your head quickly from right to left and back again. Carry out these side tilting movements for 30 to 60 seconds.

Note: It is important to make sure that you only ever tilt your head as far as feels comfortable for you. You can always build up the range and speed of the movement gradually.

Optional variations for the basic exercises

If you want to make the exercises more challenging, one option is to gradually make your stance narrower while you do them. Once you've got the hang of using the basic exercises to stimulate your vestibular system, try them out in a narrow stance or tandem stance. You will already be familiar with both of these positions from the balance assessments (pages 47 and 48–49). You can also try doing the exercises while walking forwards and backwards.

These advanced variations mix things up a bit and make your training more creative. Your brain has to keep adapting to the new, more complex versions of the exercise, which challenges your vestibular system even more and enhances the effects of the training, keeping your brain active and healthy.

Vestibulo-ocular reflex cancellation (VOR-C)

Another skill that is controlled by your vestibular system is your capacity to simultaneously accelerate and coordinate the movements of your head and eyes, keeping them in synchronisation with one another. In order to ensure the best possible coordination between your vestibular system, head, neck and eye movements, your central nervous system has to be able to suppress or 'cancel' an important vestibular reflex. The name of the following group of exercises is 'VOR-C', whereby 'VOR' stands for 'vestibulo-ocular reflex' and the 'C' stands for 'cancellation'. We'll start by showing you a simple warm-up exercise that will make it easier for you to get to grips with the more complex 'classic VOR-C' exercise that will come after.

❯ VOR-C exercises with full body rotation

VOR-C requires complex coordination of the vestibular system with movements of the eyes, head, neck and cervical spine. In order to master this skill, you can start with VOR-C full body rotations or 'spins' as a warm-up. The initial aim is to maintain a clear visual focus while you turn on the spot or swivel on a chair, without the additional challenge of coordinating your neck and cervical spine. In the next step, which is the classic VOR-C exercise, you will add in the movements of your head and cervical spine.

1. Stand with your feet hip-width apart. Lengthen your spine but keep it nice and relaxed. Allow your breath to flow smoothly and evenly. Your body should be relaxed. From this position, roll in your head and lower your nose slightly by 2 or 3 cm and lift your arms so that they are level with your eyes. Your fingers should be folded into your palms, your thumbs pointing upwards and your elbows straight. With a relaxed gaze, focus on one of your thumbnails.
2. a–e Start by turning to the right two to five times on your own axis. While you're rotating, try to keep a clear and stable view of your thumbnail, making sure that your head doesn't move and keeping your arms outstretched at eye level. Then change sides and rotate to the left. Try making the target of your focus smaller each time, switching from your thumbnail to a tiny wrinkle on your thumb. You could also try using a VisionStick (pages 78–79).

Note: This exercise might make you feel dizzy at first. That's why you should build up the speed of your rotations nice and slowly. Don't push yourself too hard. If it helps, feel free to do the exercise with your feet further apart or while sitting on a swivel chair. If you're really struggling with the exercise, start with a half or quarter turn.

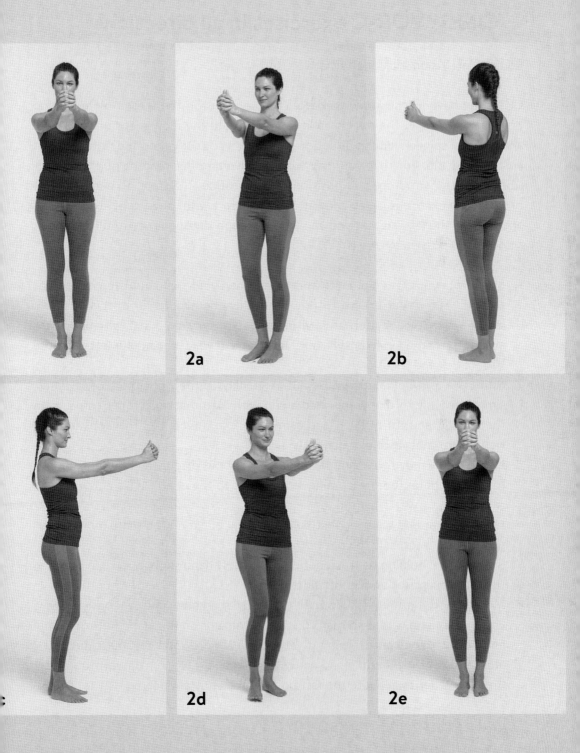

2a

2b

2d

2e

❯ Classic VOR-C exercises in all directions

Equipment: VisionStick or alternative visual target

Once you have learned how to keep a stable focus on the target while turning on your body's axis, the next step is to incorporate the movement of your head and cervical spine, in all the directions important for activating the right and left vestibular ducts. For this, you may wish to have another read through the section about the structure and position of the vestibular system on page 65. The order of the exercises is designed so that you start with movements to the right and then to the left, so that you can work through the sequence of directions as smoothly as possible.

1. Stand with your feet hip-width apart. Lengthen your spine but keep it nice and relaxed. Allow your breath to flow smoothly and evenly. From this position, hold a VisionStick or alternative visual target in your right hand, with your right arm outstretched in front of your face at eye level. Choose one letter on the VisionStick and focus on it.
2. Move the arm holding the VisionStick quickly to the right four to six times, simultaneously turning your head along with it so that your focus remains on the stick. Then return slowly and calmly back to the centre. This activates the right horizontal vestibular duct.
3. Now, quickly move your right arm, head and focus diagonally to your top right four to six times, before coming slowly back to the centre. This activates the right posterior vestibular duct.
4. Activate your left superior vestibular duct by repeating the same motion four to six times diagonally to your bottom right.
5. Switch sides, holding the VisionStick in your left hand so that you can perform the same exercises on the left side.
6. Move your left arm quickly to the left four to six times, simultaneously turning your head along with it so that your focus remains on the stick. Return calmly and slowly to the centre. This activates the left horizontal vestibular duct.
7. Now move your left arm, head and focus diagonally to your top left four to six times, in order to activate the left posterior vestibular duct.

8. Now move your left arm, head and focus diagonally to your bottom left four to six times, in order to activate the right superior vestibular duct.

Note: Keep your nose and eyes in line with the VisionStick or visual target at all times. When you first start, you will probably find that your hand moves faster and further than your head and nose do. This brings your eyes, nose and hand out of alignment. At the beginning, therefore, only move your arms to the extent and speed that still allows you to keep your nose and head in line with the target. Your

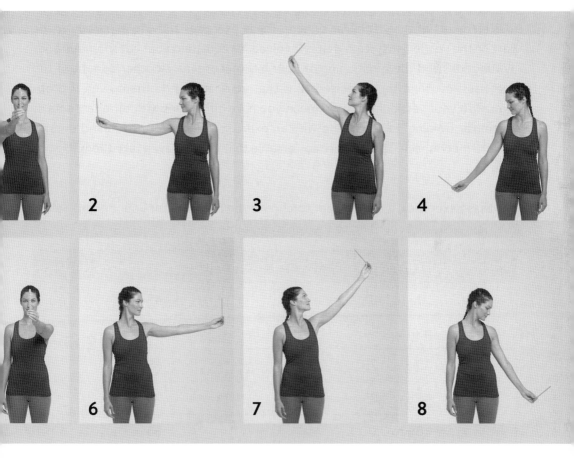

eyes should stay in a neutral position and your nose should move in line with the visual target. You can gradually build up the range and speed of the movement as you practise.

Complex vestibular exercises on the exercise ball

Large exercise balls (also known as yoga balls or Swiss balls) were originally intended for rehabilitation and vestibular training. These exercises will therefore take you back to the original purpose of this highly effective training apparatus. Exercise balls offer many different options for both training and integrating various elements of the vestibular system. These exercises activate in particular the part of the vestibular system that is involved in regulating your autonomous bodily functions and the functioning of your internal organs. Another benefit of the exercises involving the exercise ball is that you can still do them even if problems with your vestibular system mean you have difficulties with other aspects of vestibular training. Plus, training with an exercise ball is a lot of fun and doesn't require much space. The balls are so versatile that you can even take them to work with you.

For these exercises, it's important to choose the right ball for your height. Select the right ball size according to the following table.

Height in metres (m)	Diameter in centimetres (cm)
Up to 1.40	45
1.41 to 1.54	55
1.55 to 1.75	65
1.76 to 1.85	75
1.86 to 2.00	85
2.01 to 2.15	95

› Bouncing on an exercise ball

Equipment: Exercise ball

One of the easiest and most basic exercises that you can do to train the essential part of your vestibular system and activate the insular cortex is to move your body up and down at speed. This sort of vertical acceleration is perceived by the otolith organs – the saccule, to be precise – and communicated with the brain. When it receives the information regarding the acceleration, the brain initiates necessary adjustments to the spine, head and neck position as well as to the autonomous functions and the stability of the eyes. By doing this, the brain regulates the best possible posture and bodily functions for the given situation. Bouncing on an unstable surface also requires you to engage other parts of your body required for stabilisation, namely your core muscles and spine. This makes the exercise even more effective, as it activates another important part of your brain – the central section of your cerebellum. This ultimately improves the functioning of your vestibular system and makes it even more efficient.

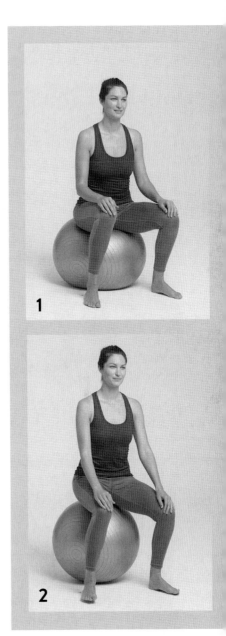

1

2

1. Sit on the exercise ball, positioning yourself in the middle. Lengthen your spine but keep it nice and relaxed with your body as relaxed as possible. Allow your breath to flow smoothly and evenly. Place your feet far enough apart to ensure you feel comfortable. Relax your face, eyes and neck.
2. Now begin to bounce gently up and down on the ball for 30 to 60 seconds. Make sure that you feel safe and comfortable with the movements. Adjust your bouncing speed and momentum as necessary.

❯ Variation 1: Bouncing on an exercise ball with eyes closed

Equipment: Exercise ball

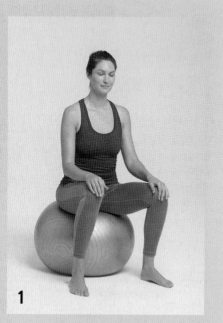

1

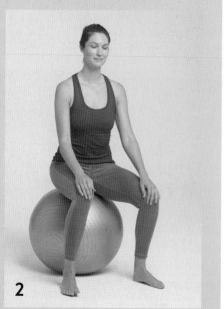

2

Once you have gotten used to bouncing on the exercise ball, you can try it with your eyes closed. As you have already seen with the 'yes-yes' and 'no-no' movements (pages 66–69 and 70–73), closing your eyes makes your brain more reliant on your vestibular system and increases the focus and efficiency of the exercise.

Note: Before you start, make sure that there's enough space around you to safely carry out the exercise with your eyes closed.

1. Sit on the exercise ball, positioning yourself in the middle. Lengthen your spine but keep it nice and relaxed with your body as relaxed as possible. Allow your breath to flow smoothly and evenly. Place your feet far enough apart to ensure you feel comfortable, and close your eyes.
2. Now begin to bounce gently up and down on the ball for 30 to 60 seconds. Make sure that you feel safe and comfortable with the movements. Adjust your bouncing speed and momentum as necessary.

❯ Variation 2: Bouncing on an exercise ball with a clear visual target

Equipment: Visual target on the wall, exercise ball

This exercise is similar to the last one, except that, with this variation, you fix your gaze on a visual target. The ability to stabilise your eyes while your body is moving is, as mentioned previously, an extremely important aspect of vestibular training. Try to keep your vision as clear and stable as possible while you're bouncing up and down – this helps to train the otolith system.

1. Sit on the exercise ball, positioning yourself in the middle. Lengthen your spine but keep it nice and relaxed with your body as relaxed as possible. Allow your breath to flow smoothly and evenly. Focus your gaze on a visual target, positioned in front of you, roughly at eye level. Make sure that you can see the visual target clearly and that it's not blurred. Place your feet far enough apart to ensure you feel comfortable.

2. Start to bounce up and down on the ball and continue to do so for 30 to 60 seconds. Make sure that you have a clear, focused view of the visual target throughout the whole exercise, and that your spine stays nice and long. Adjust your bouncing speed and momentum as necessary.

Note: In order to make them even more varied, you can also vary the direction of the momentum when doing these exercises, for example by making your upwards movements faster and your downwards movements more controlled, or vice versa.

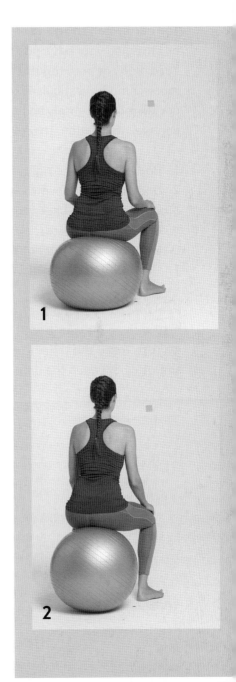

❯ Variation 3: Bouncing on an exercise ball with different postural and head positions

Equipment: Exercise ball

You can switch things up and challenge your vestibular system even more simply by changing your basic position on the exercise ball, for example by rotating your head, body or both together, or by tilting or leaning forwards or backwards. These more complex vestibular exercises are really important for activating your insular cortex more intensely and making more of an impact on how you process interoceptive information. The following head and body positions work particularly well:

1. Body tilted to the right.
2. Body tilted to the left.
3. Body extended backwards.
4. Body tilted forwards.
5. Head turned to the right.
6. Head turned to the left.

Feel free to do your preferred combination of these elements, so for example you may wish to tilt your body to the right while turning your head to the left. If you want to make the training even more challenging, you can also try transitioning smoothly between the different positions while bouncing on the ball.

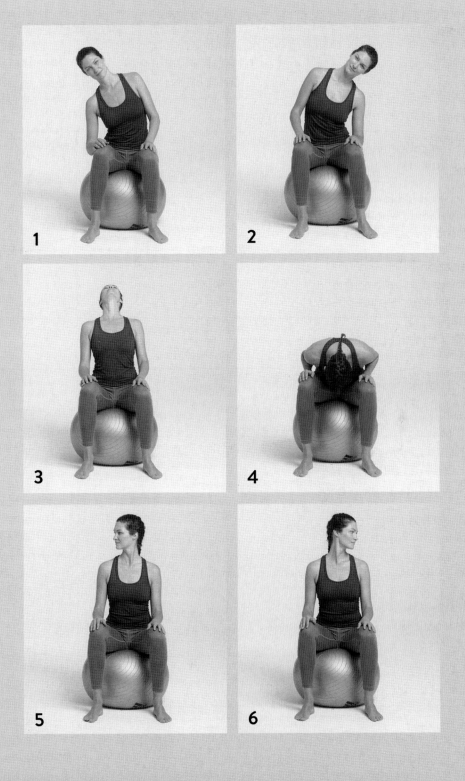

Categorising the vestibular exercises			
Exercise	Positive	Neutral/moderately positive	Save for later
Seven basic vestibular training exercises			
'No-no' movements (horizontal) (pages 66–67)			
Variation 1: 'No-no' movements with eyes closed (pages 67–68)			
Variation 2: 'No-no' movements with a clear visual target (pages 68–69)			
'Yes-yes' movements (vertical) (pages 70–71)			
Variation 1: 'Yes-yes' movements with eyes closed (pages 71–72)			
Variation 2: 'Yes-yes' movements with a clear visual target (pages 72–73)			
Lateral head tilts (pages 74–75)			
Vestibulo-ocular reflex cancellation (VOR-C)			
VOR-C exercises with full body rotation (pages 76–77)			
Classic VOR-C exercises in all directions (pages 78–79)			

Categorising the vestibular exercises			
Exercise	Positive	Neutral/moderately positive	Save for later
Complex vestibular exercises on the exercise ball			
Bouncing on an exercise ball (page 81)			
Variation 1: Bouncing on an exercise ball with eyes closed (page 82)			
Variation 2: Bouncing on an exercise ball with a clear visual target (page 83)			
Bouncing on an exercise ball with different postural and head positions (pages 84–85)			
Body tilted to the right			
Body tilted to the left			
Body extended backwards			
Body bent forwards			
Head turned to the right			
Head turned to the left			

Recommendations for vestibular training

As with the frontal lobe exercises, training the vestibular system creates a vital basis for almost all the processes that take place in your body and central nervous system. Furthermore, the vestibular system transmits a vast quantity of important information to the insular cortex. Vestibular training is therefore one of the most important tools we can give you to improve your interoceptive awareness.

Vestibular exercises as the main element of your training

You may wish to start by using the vestibular exercises as standalone training for the first three to six weeks, spending 15 to 20 minutes on them each day. This will help to develop your vestibular system and allow your insular cortex to reach a whole new level of activity and functionality. By training and developing the vestibular system, you trigger intensive activation of the posterior and central sections of the insular cortex. This also makes the integration of the other elements of interoception more effective and more sustainable, thus improving the overall framework conditions.

As a general rule, you can do the vestibular exercises in whichever order suits you best. However, we do recommend that you start with exercises that give you a good foundation for further training of this vital system. The three basic exercises – 'no-no' movements (pages 66–67), 'yes-yes' movements (pages 70–71) and lateral head tilts (pages 74–75) – are ideal for this purpose. Adjust the intensity of these exercises so that they give you positive assessment results. These simple, basic movements are all you need to get started with activating the vestibular organs. You should try to train for at least 15 to 20 minutes each day, ideally spread across two or three sessions over the course of the day.

If you're already a bit of a dab hand or vestibular training simply doesn't present too much of a challenge for you, you are more than welcome to mix things up a bit, combining exercises designed to train the different elements of your vestibular system. You can use any of the exercises from this chapter for this. One important objective of vestibular training is to return the body and brain to a state in which they can control even complex movements at all levels without excessive stress.

Because all the components of the vestibular system are responsible for delivering important information, you should attempt to have control over all aspects of the vestibular system at all times, and to incorporate them into your training. To achieve this, you can divide the exercises into small blocks, focusing on one specific aspect for two days, and then another aspect for the next two days, and so on. Tongue exercises also offer an effective way to prepare the vestibular system for further training. To do this, you can select two tongue exercises of your choice (page 191 onwards) and one to two air hunger drills (page 154 onwards), both of which will be described later in the book. One or two rounds per day of these preparatory exercises is plenty. This shouldn't take up any longer than 1 or 2 minutes of your time.

Vestibular training as part of interoceptive awareness training

Vestibular training can also be used as a building block for your overall interoceptive awareness training. Use the exercises for which you got a positive assessment result to activate your vestibular system three or four times across a day. Spend 1 or 2 minutes on each one, so that your total training time adds up to 20 to 30 minutes.

Vestibular training as a warm-up exercise

The vestibular system supports all the systems that are important for controlling movement, as well as the functionality of the central nervous system, and also intensely activates both posterior sections of the insular cortex. This makes these exercises ideal for using as a preparatory measure for interoceptive awareness training. To do this, choose one or two vestibular exercises for which you had a particularly positive assessment result and spend 30 to 90 seconds on these before commencing training on other elements of interoceptive awareness, such as respiratory training.

Recommendations for vestibular training		
Potential use	**Scope and application**	**Effect**

As the main element of the training	• Exercises with a positive or neutral/moderately positive assessment result
	• Start with the basic exercises
	• 15 to 20 minutes each day
	• In 2 to 3 sessions throughout the day
	• Carried out over the course of 3 to 6 weeks
		• Activates the posterior and central sections of the insular cortex
		• Improves:
		  • chronic pain
		  • interoceptive awareness
		  • general wellbeing and fitness
		  • digestive disorders
		  • emotional regulation

As part of interoceptive awareness training	• Exercises with positive assessment results • 1 to 2 minutes • 3 to 4 times per day	
As a warm-up for other training exercises	• 1 to 2 exercises with positive assessment results • 30 to 90 seconds • Immediately before carrying out further training	• Improves the integration of information and makes the overall training more effective

Using smell and taste to improve sensory integration

As already mentioned in Chapter 1, sensory information passes through your insular cortex from the posterior section, through the central section and into the anterior section. The sequence of activation for this vital part of the brain is therefore from back to front. The posterior section receives and calibrates sensory information; the central section integrates the information and the anterior section assigns cognitive, social and emotional components.

If we look more closely at the central section, whose role it is to integrate all the sensory information, we see that it contains special nuclei (nerve centres), which are responsible for our perception of smell and taste, as well as their intensity. What this means for you is that, by consciously discerning between different smells and tastes, you can target this specific part of the brain that is so important for integration. Differentiating between different smells and tastes is therefore a great way to prepare for training the various elements of your interoceptive awareness. On this basis, there is a range of smell and taste exercises that you should do. Not only will this help you to train both of these senses, it will also activate the functional area of the insular cortex and improve the integration of sensory information. This, in turn, will make your training more effective overall.

Sensory stimulation for weight loss

Your appetite and eating habits are dependent on a vast quantity of sensory information. The brain often uses eating as a strategy to compensate for a lack of important sensory information. Above all, the smell, taste and feel of food in your hand and mouth are important stimuli for your brain. If there is a lack of sensory stimulation in your everyday life, then when you eat, you will only feel satisfied when you have achieved sufficient stimulation from the smell, taste and feel of the food in your hand and mouth – irrespective of your actual hunger level.

If your aim is to lose weight, then as well as stimulating the tongue (pages 186–188), you should also do a short smell and taste exercise before every meal. This allows you to give your brain enough sensory stimulation without ingesting too many calories. This will help you to normalise your appetite and eating habits.

The significance of smells

Unfortunately, many people don't appreciate how important our sense of smell is. And yet, our sense of smell informs many of the vital decisions we make. It allows us to determine whether what we're smelling is dangerous, for example, or if it's good, pleasant and familiar. Our sense of smell also plays a part in choosing a partner and helps us to decide who we like and find attractive. Our sense of smell is closely connected to our sense of taste and eating habits, as well as to our memories and emotions. Olfactory information is absorbed by the odour receptors and then transported directly to the brain via the olfactory nerve (cranial nerve I). When it reaches the brain, the central section of the insular cortex is one of the regions that is responsible for processing and integrating the information. This plays an especially important role when it comes to classifying the intensity of an odour.

⟩ Differentiating and identifying smells

Material: Various small fragrance containers containing pure essential oils

When you first start your olfactory training, we recommend covering a wide range of different smells. We find that pure essential oils work well. Start by using smells that you can clearly differentiate from one another. At first, pick one earthy, one floral, one woody, one sweet and one bitter smell. Once you've become adept at identifying different categories of smells, we recommend you have a go at differentiating them even more precisely. For example, you could try to differentiate between the smells of different citrus fruits or different coniferous plants such as pine, fir and juniper. Be creative, mix things up, keep an open mind and have fun. Your brain loves new stimuli!

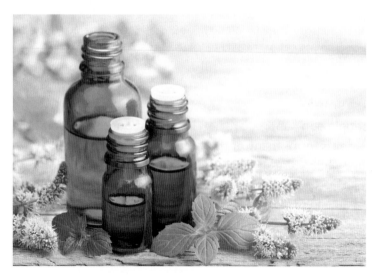

Start by choosing a range of smells that you can easily differentiate, such as lemon, pine and peppermint.

1. Prepare several small bottles with pure essential oils of different fragrances. You can be standing or sitting for this one. Lengthen your spine but keep it nice and relaxed. Allow your breath to flow smoothly and evenly. Close your eyes. Press your left index finger against your left nostril to close it and breathe the smell in through your right nostril. Breathe nice and softly through your nose and let the smell rise into your right nostril. How intensely can you smell the fragrance? Can you identify the smell? Does the smell conjure any specific memories or emotions for you? Breathe in the smell for 4 to 5 seconds and then remove it from your nostril. Repeat the process two to four times, one after the other.

2. Change sides, holding your right index finger against your right nostril to close it, and carry out the exercise with your left nostril. On which side do you notice the smell more quickly, intensely and clearly? Next, select another smell and do the exercise again with this one, first on the right and then on the left. You can use up to three different smells for your daily olfactory training. Are there certain scents that you find really difficult to smell? Or are there

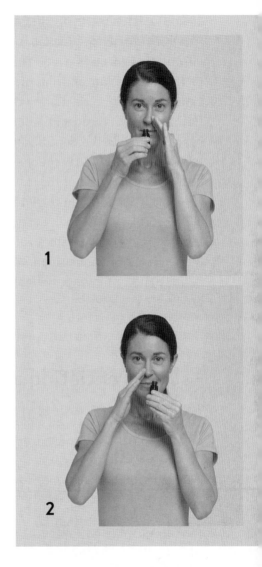

certain smells that you can't recognise or identify? Incorporate these smells into your olfactory training with increased frequency.

Make sure your training works for you

If there's a certain smell that you just really don't like, simply leave it out. It is perfectly fine to start with a palate of fragrances that you find pleasant or at least neutral.

The significance of taste

As with your sense of smell, the insular cortex also plays a significant role in the processing and integration of taste. Information relating to different flavours is integrated and processed in special nuclei in the central section of the insular cortex. As mentioned previously, this is the part of the insular cortex that is responsible for integrating all sensory information. Carrying out the recommended taste exercises is a direct way of minimising integration deficits and optimising the integration process.

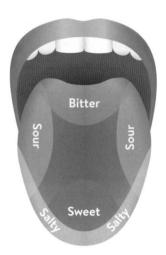

The receptors for the tastes 'sweet', 'salty', 'bitter' and 'sour' are concentrated on different areas of the tongue.

❯ Differentiating and identifying tastes

Equipment: Water-based solutions containing flavours from the categories 'sweet', 'salty', 'sour' and 'bitter'; a pipette

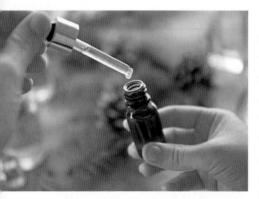

Use a pipette to apply a droplet of the solution onto the tongue.

Looking at the layout of the taste receptors for sweet, sour, bitter and salty, you can see that there are specific receptors for each taste on specific parts of the tongue. You can use this anatomical fact to give more focus to your gustatory training. As you did with the olfactory exercises, use the taste exercises to see if you can notice any differences between the left and right side of the tongue, and if one side is better at perceiving and differentiating different tastes.

1. Pick one solution flavoured with something from one of the four specified categories – 'sweet', 'sour', 'bitter' and 'salty'. Sit or stand in a comfortable position. Lengthen your spine but keep it nice and relaxed. Make sure your face, jaw and tongue are relaxed, and allow your breath to flow smoothly and evenly. Use the pipette to apply a drop of the solution to just the right-hand side of your tongue to start with, and pay attention to the flavour you can taste there. Don't worry about trying to apply the solution to the area where the specific taste buds are. It's fine simply to drip it onto the corresponding side of the tongue and then let it run along the length of your tongue. How clearly and strongly can you taste the flavour you picked?

2. Drip the same flavour onto the left side of your tongue. Pay attention to the flavour on the left-hand side and compare the clarity and intensity of the taste to that of the right-hand side. Move on to the next taste category and continue with the exercise as described, testing the right-hand side first, followed by the left-hand side. This way, you can test the different areas of the tongue one after the other and work out which side, which area and which taste buds, if any, need more training.

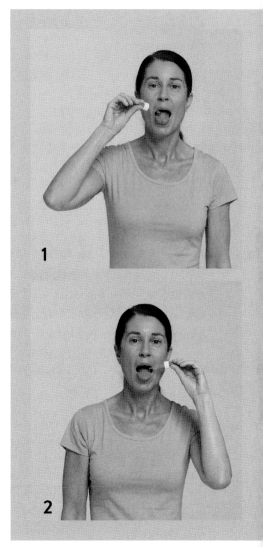

Note: As an alternative to the water-based solutions, you could work with foods that you find easy to identify. For example, you may wish to use differently flavoured sweets or any other type of food that is easy to place and move around on the tongue. Test your ability to recognise and identify the taste, as well as the intensity of the flavour – first on the right-hand side and then on the left-hand side. Give yourself the chance to identify any sensory deficits and focus your training on those areas.

Categorising the exercises for differentiating smell and taste			
Exercise	Positive	Neutral/moderately positive	Save for later
Differentiating and identifying smells (pages 92–93)			
Differentiating and identifying tastes (pages 94–95)			

Recommendations for smell and taste training

When incorporated into your overall interoceptive awareness training, smell and taste exercises work well to improve your overall interoceptive awareness. Because the central section of the insular cortex also communicates with the amygdala – the part of the brain that deals with emotions – training both of these senses has a significant positive impact on your emotional regulation. It also helps to combat digestive disorders and unhelpful eating habits. It takes very little preparation and effort to enjoy these benefits – all you have to do is work on your sense of taste for 2 or 3 minutes, three to five times a day.

Because the smell and taste training activates the central section of your insular cortex and thus improves its overall capacity for integration, one of the most effective ways of using this training is as a warm-up for other exercises. To do this, stimulate your sense of smell or taste for 1 or 2 minutes before moving on to your main training.

Another very simple option that we'd recommend is to pay more attention to your sense of smell and taste as part of your daily routine. Every meal time, take a minute to focus your awareness on the smell and taste of the food. This way, you can improve your interoceptive skills without much effort at all.

Recommendations for smell and taste training		
Potential use	Scope and application	Effect

As part of interoceptive awareness training	• 1 to 2 exercises with positive assessment results
	• 3 to 5 times per day
	• 2 to 3 minutes incorporated into your daily routine
		• Activates the central section of the insular cortex
		• Improves:
		  • digestive disorders
		  • emotional regulation
		  • healthy eating habits and normal appetite

As a warm-up for other training exercises	• 1 to 2 exercises with positive assessment results • 1 to 2 minutes • Immediately before carrying out further training	• Activates the central section of the insular cortex • Improves the integration of sensory information and makes the overall training more effective
Integration into daily routine	• Every meal time, spend 1 minute focusing your attention on the smell and taste of the food	• Supports healthy eating habits • Helps encourage a normal appetite

Preparing the vagus nerve neuromechanically

Wherever information is received, transmitted, processed and integrated within the brain, there is always the possibility that information can be lost. The majority of the interoceptive awareness exercises introduced in this book focus on the different sensory systems and their receptors, aiming to improve the way we receive information from our body and our surroundings, as well as to activate specific parts of the brain, improving their functionality. Alongside the neural aspects, certain mechanical aspects also play an important role.

As you know from reading Chapter 1, not only is the vagus nerve the most important nerve in the parasympathetic nervous system, it is also the longest nerve in the human body. It covers a wide area as it makes its way through the body, passing through several joints, various tissue structures, the diaphragm and winding its way around the internal organs. The fact that this nerve is so far-reaching means that its neuromechanical conditions can easily become impaired. It can quickly become trapped or compressed, which renders it unable to deliver information effectively to and from the affected areas. That's why it's essential, before you begin your training, to ensure that this nerve is able to travel freely through the body and carry information as effectively as possible.

In the following section, we will be showing you a series of exercises that you can do to mobilise the vagus nerve and stretch it slightly, which will optimise the quality of the neural tissue and help repair any adhesions, compressions or entrapment. One crucial mechanical factor that mustn't be overlooked is the movement of the cervical spine. Mobility deficits, particularly in the upper part of the cervical spine, can quickly cause problems with the vagus nerve.

Mobilising the cervical spine

If you look at the course of the vagus nerve and the points at which it exits the skull, you will see that it emerges from the foramen, a small opening on the underside of the skull, above the cervical spine. This is a point at which it can easily become blocked. The mobility of the first joints it comes to – the upper joints of the cervical spine – is therefore of particular importance. The diaphragmatic nerve, which is crucial to the movement of the diaphragm and the respiratory system, also emerges from the third to fifth segment of the cervical spine. This is therefore another section that we need to keep mobile and flexible, if we are to maintain the best neuromechanical conditions possible to support our respiratory system.

Mobilising the cervical spine also has a range of positive effects on both the visual and the vestibular system. It improves the transmission of information from the cervical spine to the vestibular nuclei, thus optimising the vestibulo-ocular reflexes and the control of the eyes. The following two mobilisation exercises specifically improve the mobility and posture of the cervical spine.

❯ Pushing the cervical spine backwards

The most important exercise, which has the greatest impact on the functioning of the vagus nerve and the improvement of our interoceptive accuracy, is sliding or pushing the vertebrae of the cervical spine backwards. Since we often find it easier to learn a new movement when using an external 'target', we are going to show you how to use the correct finger positioning to create a good, clear target for your movement.

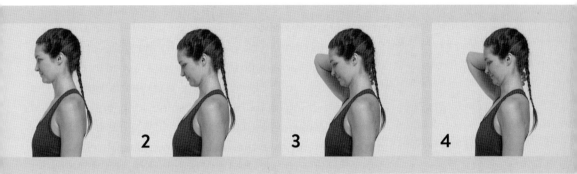

1. Sit or stand in a comfortable position. Lengthen your spine but keep it nice and relaxed. Allow your breath to flow smoothly and evenly.
2. From this position, tuck your chin slightly while lengthening your neck so that your nose and chin are lowered by 3 or 4 cm.
3. Reach your fingers behind you and place them on the centre of your cervical spine. Make sure that you can feel the little protrusions on your vertebrae with your finger tips. If you want to make the movements even easier, try rubbing your spine with your finger tips for a few seconds.
4. Now push your head and cervical spine back against your fingers in a straight line, so that your chin really pushes into your neck, forming a double chin. Then return to the starting position. Try to stay loose and relaxed throughout. Make sure that your head stays slightly rolled in the whole time. Carry out this movement four to six times consecutively. Feel free to repeat this exercise for two or three rounds.

❯ Light stretching of the cervical spine

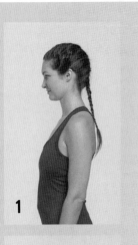

1

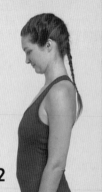

2

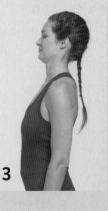

3

The second exercise improves the elongation of your entire cervical spine, which reduces the risk of mechanical obstructions of the vagus nerve or the diaphragmatic nerve. As with the previous exercise, in which you slid your upper cervical spine backwards, this exercise also benefits your visual and vestibular systems.

1. Sit or stand in a comfortable position. Lengthen your spine but keep it nice and relaxed. Allow your breath to flow smoothly and evenly.
2. From this position, tuck your chin slightly while lengthening your neck so that your nose and chin are lowered by 3 or 4 cm.
3. Now stretch your cervical spine backwards slightly. The important thing is to keep the spine long and the head rolled in. Make sure that your cervical spine is stretched out evenly and that there aren't any 'kinks'. It will take a few attempts to get used to coordinating this movement. Carry out this movement four to six times consecutively. Feel free to repeat this exercise for two or three rounds.

Note: It can be useful to combine this exercise with the previous exercise. To do so, simply return to the starting position once you've done the first exercise, and transition smoothly into the second exercise from there.

Categorising the exercises that mobilise the cervical spine			
Exercise	Positive	Neutral/moderately positive	Save for later
Pushing the cervical spine backwards			
Light stretching of the cervical spine			

Training recommendations for mobilising the cervical spine

Exercises to mobilise the cervical spine should be carried out three to five times per day, as required, spread out across the day in sessions of 2 or 3 minutes each. As a general rule, it makes sense to do these mobilisation exercises immediately before your training and to incorporate them into your day as a way of loosening up your body at the end of the day or while you're sitting down or working on the computer for prolonged periods. Adapt the intensity of the exercises to suit your range and speed of movement, so that they feel comfortable for you and give you a positive assessment result. These exercises are particularly effective for use as a warm-up for respiratory training (page 123 onwards), vestibular training (page 66 onwards) and mobilising the vagus nerve (pages 102–103). Spend 1 to 3 minutes preparing for your training by mobilising the cervical spine.

Training recommendations for mobilising the cervical spine		
Potential use	**Scope and application**	**Effect**

As a quick way to activate the vagus nerve throughout the day	• Exercises with a positive or neutral/moderately positive assessment result
	• 2 to 3 minutes
	• 3 to 5 times per day
	• Incorporate them into your daily routine:
	  • while sitting for prolonged periods, including while at your computer
	  • at the end of the day
		• Improves the functionality of the vagus nerve and the pulmonary nerve
		• Improves conditions for the vestibular system and the visual system

As a warm-up for other training exercises	• 1 to 2 exercises with positive assessment results • 1 to 3 minutes • Immediately before carrying out further training	As a warm-up for: • vestibular training • respiratory training • mobilising the vagus nerve

Mobilising the vagus nerve

Mobilising the vagus nerve is a simple way to boost its functionality before training. The aim of this is to encourage movement between this important nerve and its surrounding tissue, which helps to minimise any compression and reduce friction in the neural tissue, meaning the nerve can transport information through the body without obstruction. The vagus nerve is arranged in pairs, branching off into the right and left-hand side of the body. The following exercise describes how to mobilise the nerve on the right-hand side of the body.

› Mobilising the vagus nerve

1. Stand with your feet hip-width apart. Lengthen your spine but keep it nice and relaxed. Allow your breath to flow smoothly and evenly. Hold onto something with your left hand to stabilise yourself. Stretch out the fingers and wrist on your right-hand side, pointing your fingers upwards.
2. Pressing through your elbow, use your shoulder joint to turn your arm outwards so that your fingers are pointing behind you.
3. Keeping your arm outstretched, lift it above your head.
4. From here, stretch your arm upwards and outwards even further, lifting your shoulder blade and pushing your arm slightly out of the shoulder socket.
5. From this position, with your head slightly rolled in tilt your spine and your head to the left so that you can clearly feel tension on your right-hand side.
6. Begin the stretch by breathing deeply into the right ribs, so that they expand three-dimensionally to the front, side and back. Hold this stretch for between four and six deep breaths. The important thing here is to maintain your posture as you breathe deeply into the rib cage, making sure you can feel a deep stretch throughout. To get used to doing this complex stretch, try repeating it two or three times in succession. Then switch over and repeat the entire process for your left-hand side.

Note: If you have difficulties with the deep breathing into your ribs, we recommend using the 3D breathing exercises on page 131 as a warm-up.

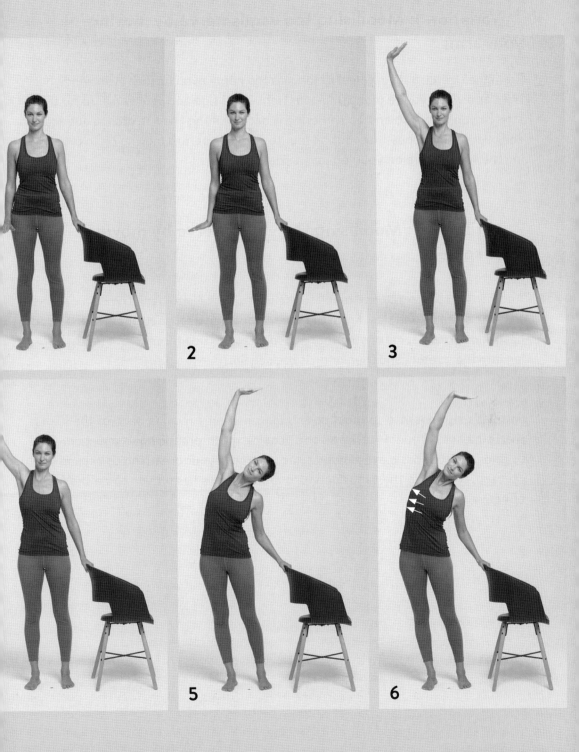

❱ Variation 1: Mobilising the vagus nerve by moving your arms

From the stretch above, you can elongate the nerve even further by moving your right arm when you're mobilising your right-hand side and vice versa. To do this, stretch your arm out and up and bring it back slightly; then stretch it out again and back again. Repeat this motion four to six times before moving on to mobilising the vagus nerve on your left-hand side.

❱ Variation 2: Mobilising the vagus nerve by moving your spine

Another way to stretch and mobilise the vagus nerve is to bend the cervical and thoracic spine to one side. From the stretch position described above, bend your head and cervical spine or your thoracic spine to the side three to five times, leaning into the stretch, and then bring it back again.

Note: It's also possible to mobilise this long nerve by moving each of the joints that it passes through. However, this requires both practice and patience. Get to grips with the basic exercise first and try to use your breathing to expand the rib cage, mobilising the vagus nerve. In practice, this has proven to be the most effective method.

Categorising the vagus nerve mobilisation exercises			
Exercise	Positive	Neutral/moderately positive	Save for later
Mobilising the vagus nerve (pages 102–103)			
Right side			
Left side			
Variation 1: Mobilising the vagus nerve by moving your arms (page 194)			
Right side			
Left side			
Variation 2: Mobilising the vagus nerve by moving your spine (page 104)			
Right side			
Left side			

Training recommendations for mobilising the vagus nerve

It is worth doing one to three short rounds of stretching to warm up the vagus nerve before going on to do other exercises to activate the vagus nerve. Mobilising the vagus nerve is particularly advisable before carrying out the breathing exercises (page 123 onwards), pressure massage (page 220) and applying heat and cold (pages 226–230), because these exercises involve the transmission of information by the vagus nerve to the insular cortex. Mobilising the vagus nerve also works wonders for coping with everyday stress. Simply do one or two rounds of one variation for which you had a particularly positive assessment result, two or three times across the day.

Training recommendations for mobilising the vagus nerve		
Potential use	**Scope and application**	**Effect**

As a quick way to activate the vagus nerve throughout the day	• 1 variation with positive assessment result
	• 1 to 2 rounds
	• 2 to 3 times per day
		• Activates the posterior section of the insular cortex
		• Improves:
		  • stress
		  • digestive disorders
		  • inflammation
		  • interoceptive accuracy

As a warm-up for other training exercises	• 1 variation with positive assessment result • 1 to 3 rounds • Immediately before carrying out further training	Particularly suitable as a warm-up for: • respiratory training • pressure massage • applying heat and cold

Activating the vagus nerve by stimulating the skin on your ear

There is one final vagus nerve activation exercise that we would recommend to give you a good basic foundation for your training. This involves direct stimulation of the vagus nerve by vibrating the area of skin inside your concha, which is innervated by the vagus nerve.

This mechanical stimulation has an overall impact on the general activity of the vagus nerve and all the systems connected to it. It also works brilliantly as a warm-up for breathing and pelvic floor exercises. We recommend using what's

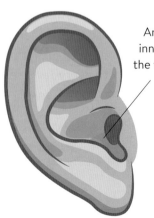

Area of skin innervated by the vagus nerve

Part of the skin on the concha is innervated by the vagus nerve and can therefore be used to activate it.

known as a 'Z-Vibe' – a small rod with a vibrating attachment made out of soft plastic. The material, size and frequency of the vibration are particularly suitable for stimulating this very sensitive area. Alternatively, you can use a simple electric toothbrush. The vibration of the handle achieves similar effects. Please be careful and make sure to place the handle on the concha, rather than in the ear canal.

❯ Sensory stimulus of the auricular branch

Equipment: Z-Vibe or small electric toothbrush

Sit or stand in a comfortable position. Lengthen your spine but keep it nice and relaxed. Allow your breath to flow smoothly and evenly. Take the Z-Vibe and turn it on to start the vibrations. Guide the tip of the Z-Vibe onto your right concha. Refer to the illustration on page 107 to see exactly where to place it. Hold the Z-Vibe so that it is gently touching the skin of the ear and vibrate for 20 to 30 seconds. Then switch sides and vibrate the inside of the left concha for 20 to 30 seconds. Feel free to do the exercise two or three times in a row. In this exercise, it's worth checking the effect it has on each side. If you get better assessment results for one side, we recommend using that side more for your training.

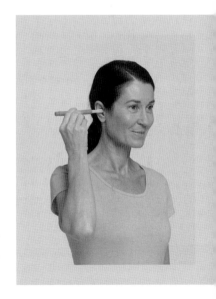

Categorising the auricular vagus nerve stimulation exercise			
Exercise	Positive	Neutral/moderately positive	Save for later
Sensory stimulus for the auricular branch (page 107)			
Right side			
Left side			
Both sides one after the other			

Training recommendations for activating the branches of the vagus nerve in the ear

You can incorporate this intensive and highly efficient exercise into your daily routine for a total of 2 to 4 minutes per day, or use it in combination with other exercises. You may find it useful to do the 'aural vibration' exercise for 1 or 2 minutes as a warm-up for further training. If you feel that it is having a positive effect, you can use vibration to stimulate the vagus nerve for 1 to 3 minutes while carrying out other training such as breathing, tongue and pelvic floor exercises. Find the right level of intensity by doing an assessment.

Training recommendations for activating the branches of the vagus nerve in the ear		
Potential use	**Scope and application**	**Effect**

As part of interoceptive awareness training	• Sensory stimulus of the auricular branch exercise with positive assessment result
	• 2 to 4 minutes each day
	• Divided into several small sessions
		• Activates the posterior section of the insular cortex
		• Improves:
		  • digestive disorders
		  • inflammation
		  • stress
		  • interoceptive awareness
		  • general wellbeing and fitness

As a warm-up for other training exercises	• Sensory stimulus of the auricular branch exercise with positive assessment result • 1 to 2 minutes • Immediately before carrying out further training	Particularly suitable as a warm-up for: • respiratory training • pelvic floor training • vestibular training

Improving bilateral movements

Certain movements, such as breathing, swallowing, speaking, humming or pelvic floor exercises, require both sides of the body to work in synchronisation with one another (bilateral movement). There is a specific part of the frontal lobe that is dedicated to preparing and coordinating these bilateral movements. This is called the supplementary motor area. It plays a particularly significant role in coordinating our breathing, as well as tongue and swallowing movements. The supplementary motor areas in each half of the frontal lobe are also heavily involved in stabilising our core, giving us a better foundation for bilateral coordination.

› Vibrating the front teeth

Equipment: Z-Vibe or electric toothbrush

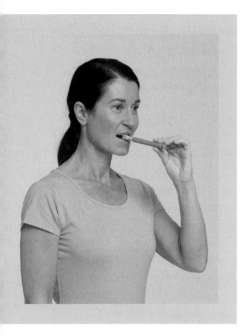

One of the fastest and most efficient methods of activating the supplementary motor area is to vibrate the front incisors. The Z-Vibe, which you will already be familiar with from stimulating the parts of the vagus nerve in the ear (sensory stimulus of the auricular branch page 107), was actually developed as a speech and language aid and is specially designed for use in the mouth – particularly for children. If you don't want to buy a Z-Vibe, you can also use an electric toothbrush or similar device. However, the Z-Vibe works particularly well for this exercise due to its surface quality, size and the frequency of the vibrations.

Sit or stand in a comfortable position. Lengthen your spine but keep it nice and relaxed. Allow your breath to flow smoothly and evenly. Turn on the Z-Vibe (or electric toothbrush) to start it vibrating and place it between your front incisors. Bite down gently so that you can feel the vibration in your teeth. Continue vibrating your teeth for about 20 seconds.

Note: If you have crowns or fillings in this section of your mouth or you find this exercise uncomfortable, try lowering the intensity by reducing the contact between the Z-Vibe and your teeth. Feel free to place your lips between the teeth and the Z-Vibe, cover the Z-Vibe with a thin cloth or use a different section of your teeth.

Bilateral hand movements

One of the most effective ways to support and improve the coordination and control of your core is through a series of complex exercises involving hand coordination. When coordinating your hand movements, your brain has to ensure maximum stability of your core. If you carry out complex movements with both hands, you activate the supplementary motor areas, which are responsible for the stabilisation and coordination of the core. Activating these areas by coordinating the hands is therefore a brilliant tool to help you prepare for tongue, breathing and pelvic floor exercises, making them easier to do.

Once you start working your way through the small selection of very effective exercises described in the following selection, you will soon see an improvement in the functioning of these supplementary motor areas and your subsequent training. The bilateral hand movements work really well in combination with dental vibration.

❭ Opening and closing the hands alternatingly

1. Stand with your feet hip-width apart. Lengthen your spine but keep it nice and relaxed. Look straight ahead with a neutral gaze. Allow your breath to flow smoothly and evenly. From this position, bend your elbows 90 degrees, so that your forearms are parallel to the floor. Stretch your right wrist and the fingers of your right hand, while simultaneously bending your left hand and curling up your fingers.

2. Now alternate between bending and stretching your wrist and fingers, so that you're pushing your wrist forward and your fingers upward with one hand, while simultaneously curling in the fingers of the other hand and bending that wrist towards the floor. Start by doing this exercise gently and slowly and gradually increase the speed as you get better at it and gain more control over the movements. The goal is to switch between the movements as quickly as possible. Carry out this exercise for 20 to 30 seconds.

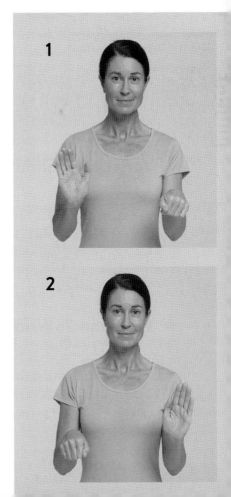

❯ Bilateral wrist rotations

Another way to stimulate the supplementary motor areas is through complex hand movements in which you move the hands in the same or opposite direction. The following describes how to do bilateral wrist rotations, where you rotate both wrists at the same time. Rather than drawing circles in the air, you can also write your name or the alphabet, or even draw a figure of eight. Essentially, you can do whatever you like, as long as you're moving both hands simultaneously in the same or opposite direction.

1–4   Stand with your feet hip-width apart. Lengthen your spine but keep it nice and relaxed. Allow your breath to flow smoothly and evenly. Look straight ahead with a neutral gaze. From this position, bend your elbows 90 degrees, so that your forearms are parallel with the floor. With your fingers closed, start circling your right hand in a clockwise direction and your left hand in an anti-clockwise direction around your wrist, which should remain in position. Keep this going for five to six rotations. Try to make the rotations the same size and speed with both hands. Switch direction and circle the right hand anti-clockwise and the left hand clockwise.

❯ Variation 1: Simultaneous rotation

To make the exercise a little more varied, you can circle both hands simultaneously clockwise and anti-clockwise. Again, you should make sure that both hands are moving at the same speed and with the same range of motion.

❯ Variation 2: Writing your name or drawing

You can also try writing your name, whole sentences or drawing shapes as a way to move your hands in parallel and in synchronisation. You can pretty much be as

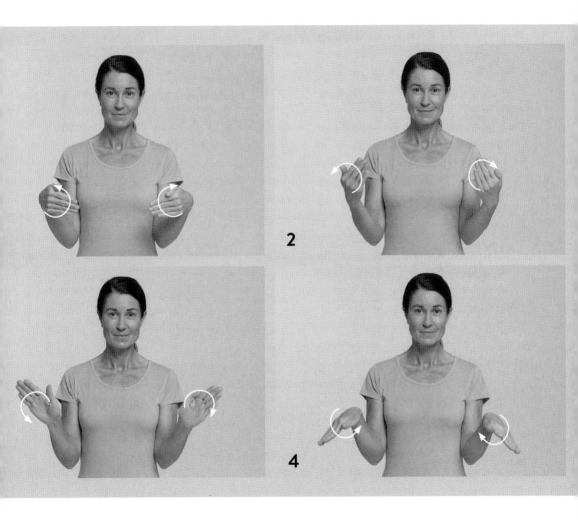

creative as you like. As an example, you could try moving your hands in opposite directions, so you write your name forwards with one hand and write the letters of your name backwards with the other. You could also try writing it to the left with one hand and to the right with the other, or move both hands from the outside in or from the inside out. Carry out this writing exercise for 20 to 30 seconds. Repeat the process two or three times, one after the other.

Categorising the exercises for activating the supplementary motor areas (simultaneous activation of both sides of the body)			
Exercise	Positive	Neutral/moderately positive	Save for later
Vibrating the front teeth (page 110)			
Alternating between opening and closing the hands (page 111)			
Bilateral wrist rotations (pages 112–113)			
Variation 1: Simultaneous rotation (page 112)			
Variation 2: Writing your name or drawing (pages 112–113)			

Training recommendations for activating the supplementary motor areas

As with activating the auricular vagus nerve, exercises that activate the supplementary motor area also work really well as a warm-up for breathing, tongue and pelvic floor exercises. To use them in this way, simply pick one or two exercises for which you had very positive assessment results, and spend 30 to 120 seconds on them before starting the next part of your training. Carrying out complex bilateral hand movements along with dental vibration is one of the most effective combinations we can recommend. Use the assessments to check which combination works best for you.

Training recommendations for activating the supplementary motor areas		
Potential use	Scope and application	Effect

As a warm-up for other training exercises	• 1 to 2 exercises with positive assessment results
	• 30 to 120 seconds each
	• Immediately before carrying out further training
	
	For the best results, combine vibrating the front teeth (page 110) with complex hand movements ('alternating between opening and closing the hands' on page 111 or 'bilateral wrist rotations' on pages 112–113).
		• Activates the posterior section of the insular cortex
		• Improves the overall effectiveness of the training
		• Improves:
		  • chronic pain
		  • pain symptoms, especially in the core
		  • pelvic floor problems
		• Particularly suitable as preparation for:
		  • respiratory training
		  • pelvic floor training
		  • vestibular training

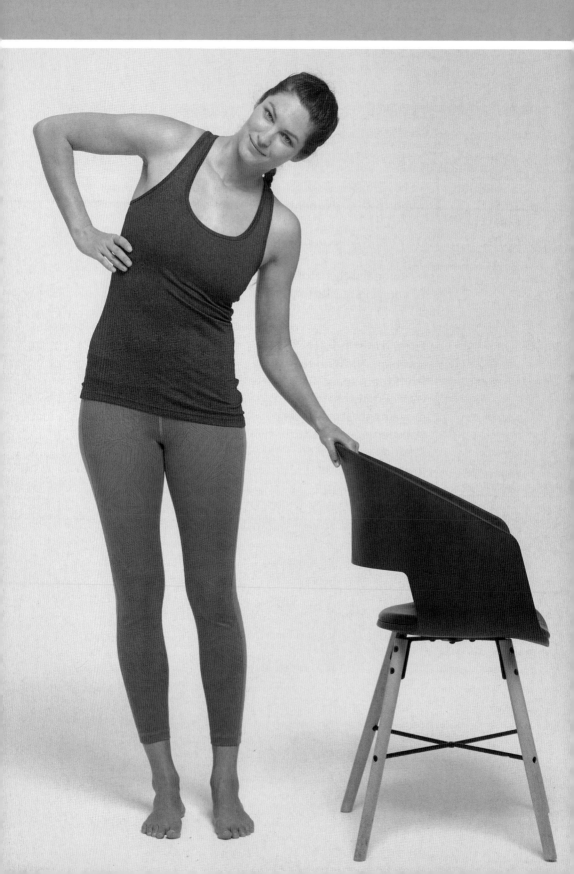

4

Breathing and the pelvic floor

The power of breathing

Many cultures around the world have acknowledged over the last few thousand years the crucial role that the right breathing techniques play in our health. Breathing is the central focus of yoga, pilates, relaxation techniques and meditation, for example. Our day-to-day vernacular is full of expressions that indicate how extremely important breathing is – we talk about how we 'live and breathe' things that are extremely important to us, for example, and encourage others to 'just breathe' when faced with adversity. Breathing is also extremely important for the brain and central nervous system. Physiologically, the brain needs two things to survive: glucose and oxygen. If there is an insufficient supply of either of these substances, this always has serious and far-reaching consequences for your health and the functioning of your brain and body. And yet, that also works the other way around, as the health and functionality of your brain, central nervous system and body affect how well you regulate your breathing.

How stress affects your breathing

From a neural perspective, there are various centres in the brain stem that initiate, coordinate and control our breathing. These centres contain special nuclei, which are responsible for initiating inhalation, prolonged exhalation and much more. Exercises specifically designed to train the respiratory system also improve the neural activity in the brain stem (pons and medulla), as well as in the midbrain, which is an additional benefit for our health.

Breathing is a largely unconscious process. It is autonomously regulated and is strongly influenced by the activity of the sympathetic and parasympathetic nervous systems. If the balance between these two important components of the autonomous nervous system is disturbed, this has a negative impact on the body and causes symptoms of stress. For example, when we are under a lot of stress our breathing becomes faster and shallower, which can affect the balance of blood gases, the pH value of the blood or its oxygen-binding capacity. Simply put: our overall health suffers.

Breathing activates the vagus nerve and restores biochemical balance

One of the most important functions of respiratory training is to counteract these negative effects on a mechanical, physiological and neural level. The average person takes between 18,000 and 20,000 breaths per day. This means that the patterns of movement we have formed are deeply ingrained in the brain and, in normal circumstances, proceed autonomously and unconsciously. Therefore, in order to make positive and sustainable changes, we have to dedicate a little more time to our breathing exercises – at least 20 to 30 minutes per day.

If we consider how closely related our breathing is to our sense of interoception, there are several important components to cover. First of all, respiration is a process that takes place inside the body and influences and regulates numerous other internal processes and functions there. The mechanical process of respiration causes the chest and abdominal cavity to move, and so the vagus nerve is activated and mobilised with every breath we take. A good breathing technique also moves and lightly massages the organs in the abdomen, which in turn stimulates our lymphatic flow. All this information is sent to the insular cortex. Our breathing technique also affects our blood pressure and initiates and regulates a range of biochemical metabolic processes.

Our breathing also causes constant changes in the composition of our blood gases. This too is information that is evaluated in the posterior section of the insular cortex. Regardless of whether our bodies need to adjust the pH value, balance out the ratio of oxygen to carbon dioxide, or break down lactic acid – breathing is key to ensuring the right balance, and is therefore one of the most important tools we have when it comes to restoring our body's biochemical balance. Furthermore, the mouth, nose and throat are involved in breathing and are therefore activated by respiratory training. This area is so important for interoceptive awareness that we have dedicated a whole chapter to it (Chapter 5, page 183 onwards). Practising good breathing techniques is one of the most important tools we have for improving our interoceptive awareness and ensuring a happy life with less stress.

Breathing exercises to target specific symptoms

For the most effective respiratory training, there are three key elements to target. We will be focusing on these elements in this chapter:

1. Improving the coordination of your respiratory muscles (page 121 onwards): The first aspect of respiratory training is all about improving the mechanics of the respiratory system, focusing on the muscles that allow us to breathe. For this, you will be doing exercises aimed at the following:
   - Optimising the movement of the diaphragm (pages 122–130)
   - Improving rib cage mobility (pages 130–137)
   - Strengthening the respiratory muscles (pages 137–142)
2. Breathing techniques to prolong exhalation (page 146 onwards): In this section, you will be learning simple techniques for prolonging your exhalation.
3. Air hunger drills (page 154 onwards): In the third section, we will be teaching you a series of exercises known as 'air hunger drills'. These are an efficient way to combat the various physiological effects caused by the way we breathe when we're stressed.

Using the different aspects of respiratory training, you can have a huge impact on the overall functionality and activity of your insular cortex. Training the mechanical components of the respiratory system has a particularly positive effect on activity levels within the posterior section of the insular cortex, which is closely related to more physical issues. For example, focused training of the respiratory system works well for those experiencing problems with their pelvic floor or digestive system, and creates a good foundation for further respiratory training. The prolonged exhalation exercises target both the posterior and anterior sections of the insular cortex by encouraging increased focus and attention. They are also very effective at alleviating pain and any issues with emotional regulation. They are a precursor to the air hunger drills described later. These exercises activate all three parts of the insular cortex, which means they also have the power to increase your capacity for integration in the central section of the insular cortex. Air hunger drills are ideal for improving your overall interoceptive awareness, as well as emotional regulation. They can also help to alleviate anxiety and chronic pain.

First, we will show you some exercises you can do to prepare for your respiratory training, which will make your training easier and more efficient. If you find the breathing exercises difficult, feel free to come back to these preparatory exercises at any time. We advise that you spend 1 to 2 minutes on these exercises before your training, as they will help to prepare and improve the functioning of the parts of the brain that coordinate your breathing. We are focusing here on the parts of the brain stem and the supplementary motor areas in the frontal lobe (page 110) that help to organise the respiratory process. In addition, it is very helpful to activate the vagus nerve specifically, because this also has a huge impact on the quality of your breathing. The easiest way to improve the function of the supplementary motor areas is through dental stimulation and, for the vagus nerve, by stimulating the skin on the concha. To do this, perform the exercises vibrating the front teeth (page 110) and sensory stimulus of the auricular branch (page 107) for 30 to 60 seconds each. Alternatively, you can improve the functioning of these areas of the brain by gargling and then swallowing water. Further information can be found in Chapter 5 'Tongue and throat' (from page 183).

Improving the coordination of the respiratory muscles

To make our respiratory training as efficient and easy as possible, it's really important that we first establish well-functioning respiratory muscles and good chest mechanics. Poor posture, illness, injury, lack of movement and activity or stress-related changes in breathing are common factors that limit the function and mobility of the respiratory muscles. As the main respiratory muscle, the diaphragm in particular is often affected. This important muscle, which attaches to the lower ribs, has fascial tissue that draws into the chest area and towards the lumbar spine. The diaphragm is by far the most active muscle in the respiratory system. It is supported by the intercostal and core muscles and, where there is a high degree of exertion, also by the auxiliary respiratory muscles. The diaphragm is mechanically and neurally connected to important areas of the mouth and throat, as well as to the pelvic floor. Improving the functioning of this vital respiratory muscle not only has a positive effect on our breathing itself, but also on the other systems that are connected to the diaphragm. For example, back pain, tension in the shoulders and neck area or pelvic floor issues are often related to poor diaphragm mobility and can be improved by focused respiratory training.

As well as making your breathing easier, lighter and more efficient, improving the coordination of your respiratory system mechanics and strengthening the respiratory muscles also increases your brain's ability to perceive and control the movements of the chest and diaphragm.

Optimising the movement of the diaphragm

If you look at the process of breathing, you will see that, when you inhale, the diaphragm contracts and moves down into the abdomen. Expanding the chest causes the lungs to fill with air. When you exhale, the diaphragm moves up towards the rib cage and lungs and relaxes. This pushes the air back out of the lungs. To stretch this muscle, you need to focus on exhaling and forcing the air out of your lungs. In the following section, we will show you a range of exercises you can use to stretch and loosen this muscle.

The basic exercise designed to reduce the amount of tension in this muscle is the diaphragm stretch, which you can achieve through intensive, prolonged exhalation. The easiest way to do this exercise is to lie down with your knees bent and your feet flat on the floor. This is the ideal position for learning how to do the stretch. Once you've mastered the exercise, you can also do it sitting or standing.

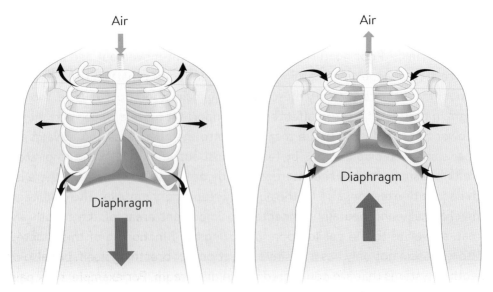

When you breathe in, your diaphragm sinks down towards your abdominal area; when you breathe out, it rises in the direction of your rib cage.

❯ Diaphragm stretch

Equipment: Mat

The main aim of the exercise is to achieve a deep stretch in the diaphragm through long, deep exhalation. It takes a little time and practice to really get the hang of allowing and controlling such a deep exhalation.

1. Lie on your back with your knees bent and your feet flat on the floor.
2. Tilt your pelvis to bring your lower spine down towards the floor, so that it lies flat against the mat.
3. Place one hand on your stomach and take three or four breaths, using your hand to feel how your abdominal wall rises and falls as you breathe.
4. Start the exercise by taking a deep breath in through your nose, if possible, inhaling right down into your stomach so that your hand and stomach rise upwards.
5. Now breathe out fully. The exhalation should be rapid and long, but controlled. Keep your throat, neck and mouth relaxed. The important thing is to have your mouth and jaw open and relaxed. Focus on the how your breath feels as it flows out of your lungs and through your mouth, and try not to force the breath out. Exhale completely. When you feel that

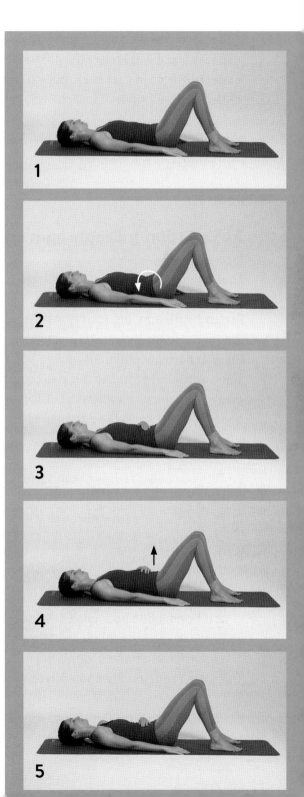

you have exhaled all the air in your lungs, breathe out a little more. Keep your pelvis and lower spine on the floor. If you're doing it properly, you should feel a deep stretch in your back, pulling upwards towards your lungs. Do this exercise three or four times consecutively, taking a little break in between each one.

Note: This stretch often makes people feel the need to cough. This is nothing to worry about. It will wear off as you practice.

❱ Variation 1: Diaphragm stretch – arms above the head

Equipment: Mat

For this variation, lift your arms over your head as you inhale, placing them on the mat, and let them relax there as you fully exhale. This arm position improves the mechanical conditions, giving you a deeper diaphragm stretch. If you aren't able to lift your arms like this due to poor shoulder mobility, start by using a small pillow or cushion to support your forearms. You will notice, however, that this will become easier too as you keep practising.

1. Lie on your back with your knees bent and your feet flat on the floor.
2. Tilt your pelvis to bring your lower spine down towards the floor, so that it lies flat against the mat.
3. Take a deep breath in through your nose, if possible, breathing right down into your stomach, raising your arms above your head as you inhale.
4. Keep your throat and neck nice and loose, with your jaw and mouth slightly open. Now begin to exhale quickly, but keeping the breath controlled and your throat, neck and mouth relaxed. Your arms should be resting gently on the floor above your head to support the diaphragm stretch. If you're doing it properly, you should feel a deep stretch in your back, pulling upwards towards your thoracic spine. Do this exercise three or four times consecutively, taking a little break in between each one.

Note: Try not to push the air into the back of your throat, and make sure that your pelvis and spine stay on the floor.

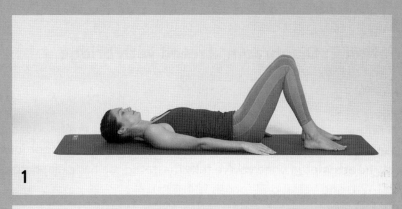

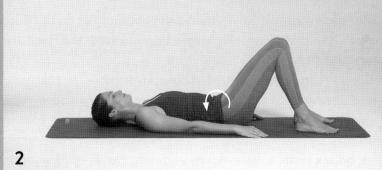

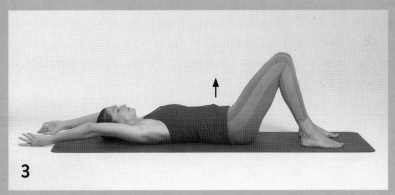

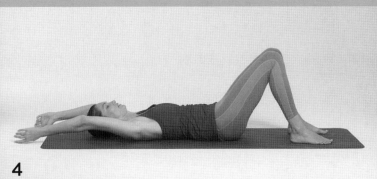

❭ Variation 2: Diaphragm stretch with bridge

Equipment: Mat

For this variation, you add in a bridge pose, which further intensifies the diaphragm stretch as you breathe out. This exercise requires quite a bit of coordination and should only be attempted once you've fully mastered the basic diaphragm stretch (pages 123–124) and Variation 1 (pages 124–125).

1. Lie on your back with your knees bent and your feet flat on the floor.
2. Tilt your pelvis to bring your lower spine down towards the floor, so that it lies flat against the mat.
3. Take a deep breath in through your nose, if possible, so that your stomach swells upwards, while simultaneously raising your arms above your head and lifting your back and pelvis off the ground. Make sure that your pelvis stays tucked in.
4. From this bridge pose, exhale rapidly and fully, but keeping your breath controlled. Your throat, neck and mouth should be relaxed.
5. Just before you finish exhaling, lower your pelvis back down to the floor as you breathe out, keeping it tucked in. This lowering motion gives your respiratory muscles an even more powerful stretch. Carry out this exercise two to four times consecutively.

Note: This variation takes a little practice to get right – have patience and practise regularly.

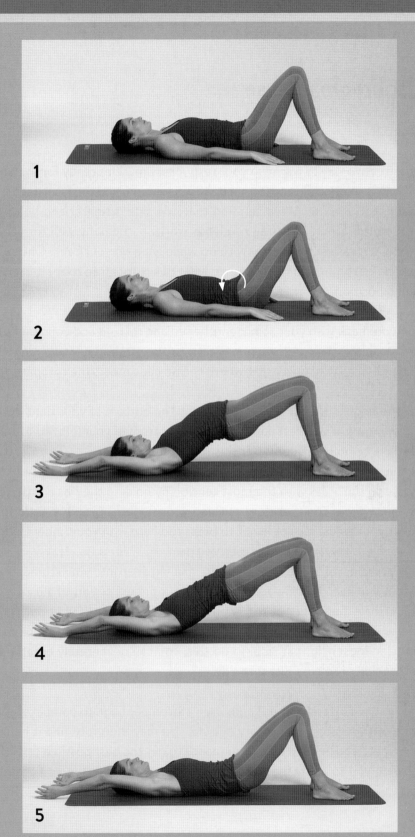

❯ Diaphragm release

Equipment: Mat

Another effective way to warm up your respiratory muscles ready for the breathing exercises is to massage and loosen up the diaphragm and the fascial structures that attach it to the ribs. We often find that one side is tighter and holds more tension than the other. Diaphragm release works particularly well for reducing this tension. It's easiest to learn how to do while lying on your back. Once you've got the hang of diaphragm release while lying down, feel free to try it in a sitting or standing position.

1. Lie on your back with your spine lengthened and relaxed and your knees bent, feet flat on the floor. Allow your breath to flow smoothly and evenly. Place your hands onto your lower ribs, where the rib cage meets the soft part of your stomach.
2. Place the fingers of your right hand around the bottom of your right outer rib and the fingers of your left hand around the bottom of your left rib. You should essentially be holding your lower ribs with your fingers.
3. Feel the tension of the respiratory muscle with your finger tips. Apply light pressure to the areas with the most tension by holding the ribs a little tighter with your fingers and therefore pushing your fingers upwards a little further towards your lungs. Take care not to press too hard with your fingers, and certainly don't do anything that causes you pain.
4. Start by taking five to ten deep breaths, inhaling deep into your stomach. Make sure that you keep holding your ribs with your fingers as you inhale.
5. As you exhale, pull your ribs firmly but gently down towards your pelvis. Try to notice which side is holding more tension. You will need to focus more on massaging and loosening that side. To do this, you can deliberately breathe more into that side or release just that side.

Note: At first, we often find our hands aren't strong enough to compete with the resistance of this strong respiratory muscle. You may therefore find it helpful to work out where you need to place your hands to get the best possible grip of your ribs, allowing you to apply the necessary counterpressure when you breathe in,

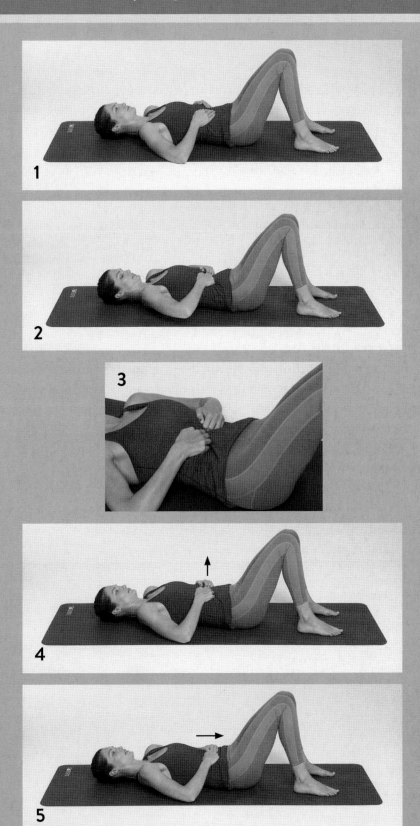

as well as to pull the ribs down towards your pelvis as you breathe out. Try experimenting a little with your grip until you find the best position. As time goes on, your hands will get stronger and you will be able to carry out the exercise for 2 to 3 minutes at a time.

Don't overdo it

This exercise shouldn't cause you too much tension, and definitely shouldn't be painful. Adjust how hard you press with your fingers and how deep your breaths are to ensure that you're working within your comfort zone.

Improving rib cage mobility

As well as improving the functioning of the diaphragm, another fundamental aspect of good breathing technique is maximum ventilation of all areas of the lung. We can achieve this by improving the three-dimensional coordination of the chest movement. By 'three-dimensional' we mean that, when we inhale, both sides of the chest should expand synchronously in three directions: forwards, sideways and backwards. If movement is restricted in any one of these directions, you need to work on this area to ensure that it is fully integrated into the breathing process. In the following section, we will show you a series of exercises you can use to specifically improve the coordination of your chest movements and the ventilation of your lungs.

〉 3D breathing

3D breathing is the easiest way to gain better awareness and control over the movement of the chest. This exercise not only helps you to guide the breath into all sections of the lungs, but also to improve the coordination and strength of the respiratory muscles that move the rib cage. In addition, it focuses your interoceptive awareness on the process of breathing.

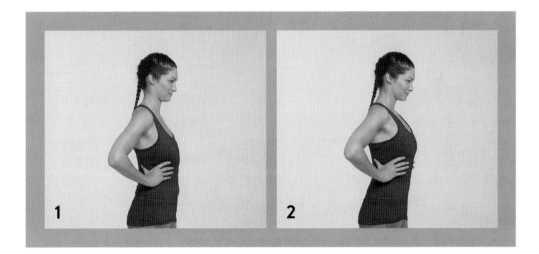

1. Stand with your feet hip-width apart. Lengthen your spine but keep it nice and relaxed. Allow your breath to flow smoothly and evenly. Place your hands on each side of your rib cage so that your thumbs are pointing backwards and your other four fingers are flat against the front of your rib cage.
2. Now take three or four deep breaths, in and out, keeping the breath soft. Pay attention to whether you feel your rib cage expanding forwards, sideways and backwards as you inhale. Notice if there are any differences between your left and right side. Are there areas that only move a little or not at all? These areas are not fully integrated into the breathing process. The next step focuses on increasing the involvement of these areas in the respiratory movement. We usually find that it's the backwards movement that is a little more limited.

〉 Activating the intercostal muscles

If the exercise above indicated that certain areas are not fully integrated into the breathing process, you should focus your attention on these areas. If you vigorously tap or slap the areas of the rib cage that don't expand as fully during 3D breathing, you will see improvements astonishingly quickly.

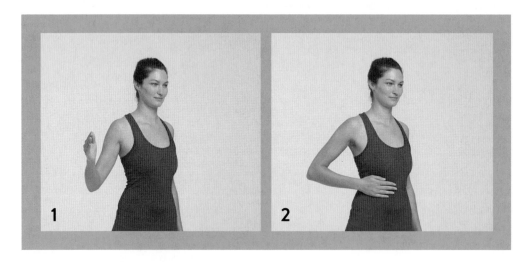

1. Stand with your feet hip-width apart. Lengthen your spine but keep it nice and relaxed. Allow your breath to flow smoothly and evenly. Focus on the area where there was inadequate movement during the 3D breathing exercise.
2. Firmly slap these parts of the rib cage two or three times with the palm of your hand. You should be able to clearly feel the tapping and it's even fine for it to be slightly uncomfortable, as long as it doesn't exceed your pain threshold. After completing this correction, repeat the 3D breathing exercise and see if you notice any changes. If necessary, repeat this exercise two or three times.

❯ **3D breathing with a side bend**

Equipment: Chair or other object to hold onto, such as a wall

Once you've mastered the 3D breathing, it's time for the next step. 3D breathing with a side bend is an excellent way to focus your attention and training on improving your breathing on one side of the body. To do this, simply carry out the 3D breathing exercise as described on page 131, but lean your body to the side and focus only on the breathing movement of the side that's open and stretched.

1. Stand with your feet hip-width apart. Lengthen your spine but keep it nice and relaxed. Allow your breath to flow smoothly and evenly. To activate the right side, hold onto the back of a chair or similar object with your left hand to steady yourself. Take two or three breaths here, paying attention to your breathing, and then bend your upper body to the left side. Make sure that your spine is lengthened and bends evenly to the side. Don't lean too far – a little bend is plenty to begin with.
2. Place your right hand on your lower right ribs.
3. Breathe in, expanding into your hand. Pay attention to how the rib cage expands to the front, side and back, pressing into your hand. Breathe consciously into your right hand for 30 to 60 seconds. Then, do the exercise on the other side, bending your body to the right instead. In this position, breathe into your left hand for 30 to 60 seconds.

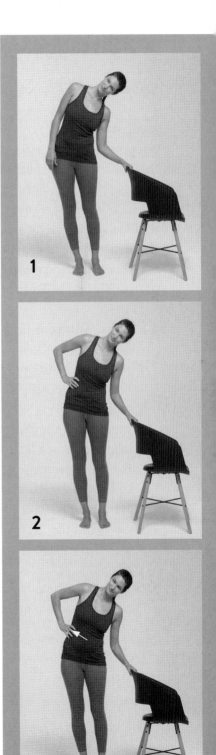

1

2

3

❭ 3D staggered breathing with a side bend

Equipment: Chair or other object to hold onto, such as a wall

If you want to make this breathing exercise a little more creative and increase its effectiveness, you can try staggering your 3D breathing with a side bend. With this exercise, you split the 3D breathing into three stages, breathing first into the lower section of the rib cage, then into the middle and then into the top. This exercise is ideal for gaining a better awareness of the respiratory movement of each half of the body and optimising the mechanical and functional elements of the diaphragm and chest movement. Above all, it will allow you to focus and control your breathing more precisely, and therefore to achieve a greater awareness of the different aspects of the breathing process.

1. a Stand with your feet hip-width apart. Lengthen your spine but keep it nice and relaxed. Allow your breath to flow smoothly and evenly. To activate the right side, hold onto the back of a chair or other object with your left hand to steady yourself. Take two or three breaths in, paying attention to your breathing, and then bend your upper body to the left side. As you do this, make sure that your spine is lengthened and bends evenly to the side. Don't lean too far – a little bend is plenty to begin with. Place your right hand on the right lower ribs.

1. b Carry out the 3D breathing exercise for two or three breaths.

2. a Place your hand on the central section of your rib cage.

2. b Carry out the 3D breathing exercise for two or three breaths.

3. a Place your hand on the upper section of your rib cage, just underneath the armpit.

3. b Breathe consciously into the upper section of your rib cage. Again, pay attention to the movement of your fingers during the 3D breathing.

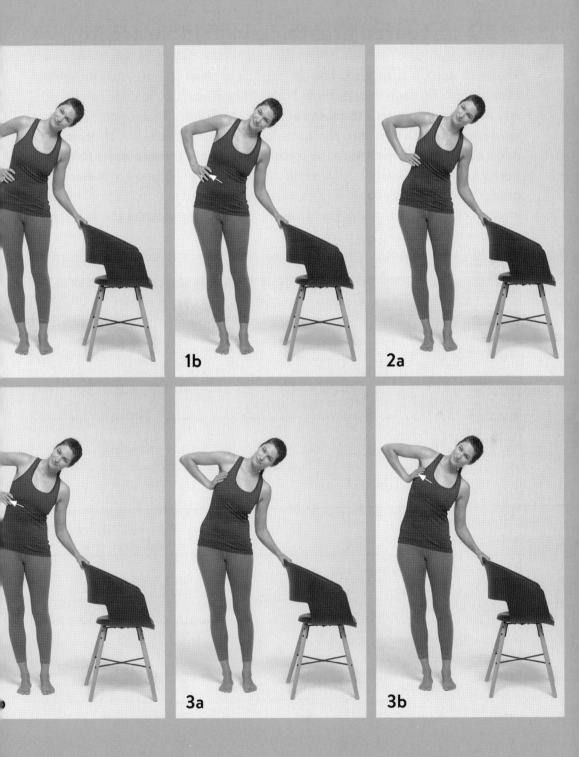

1b

2a

3a

3b

❯ 3D staggered breathing in a single breath

The next step up is to learn how to produce a three-dimensional movement of the whole rib cage in one single breath. Again, start by leaning to one side, and then use one breath to fill the whole rib cage with air, section by section. Guide your breath first into the deep lower region of the ribs, then into the middle section and finally into the top of the rib cage. The important thing is to breathe slowly and evenly, controlling the flow. Take your time and feel how the breath gradually fills your whole rib cage from the bottom to the top, expanding it in all three directions. Feel free to use your hand to feel the movement of your ribs.

Categorising the exercises for improving coordination of the respiratory muscles			
Exercise	Positive	Neutral/moderately positive	Save for later
Optimising the movements of the diaphragm			
Diaphragm stretch (pages 123–124)			
Variation 1: Diaphragm stretch – arms above the head (pages 124–125)			
Variation 2: Diaphragm stretch with bridge (pages 126–127)			
Diaphragm release (pages 128–130)			

Categorising the exercises for improving coordination of the respiratory muscles			
Exercise	Positive	Neutral/moderately positive	Save for later
Improving rib cage mobility			
3D breathing (page 131)			
Activating the intercostal muscles (page 132)			
3D breathing with a side bend (page 133)			
3D staggered breathing with a side bend (pages 134–135)			
3D staggered breathing in a single breath (page 136)			

Strengthening the respiratory muscles

As well as improving the coordination of the breathing process and the mechanics of your respiratory system, another important element is to strengthen your respiratory muscles. The better your muscles function, the easier you will find it to do the breathing exercises and to breathe in general – and the better your breathing will be. In the following section, we will show you two exercises designed to strengthen the respiratory muscles. These are advanced variations of the 3D breathing exercise. We will then show you how to work with respiratory training devices that can be used specifically to improve your respiratory muscles with regard to inhalation and exhalation.

❯ 3D breathing with a resistance band

Equipment: Resistance band

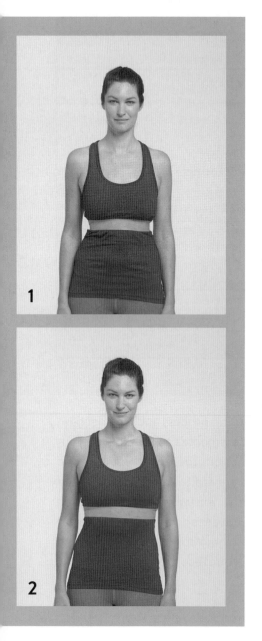

A great way to give your respiratory muscles an even more intense workout during the 3D breathing exercise and to create new stimuli is to do the exercise while using a resistance band to apply counterpressure to the rib cage as you inhale. This external resistance not only strengthens your respiratory muscles, but also helps you to increase your awareness of your breathing and the movement of your ribs. All you need for this is a short, elasticated resistance band. You can use a mini circular band or any other stretchy elasticated band that will tightly enclose your ribs.

1. Stand with your feet hip-width apart. Lengthen your spine but keep it nice and relaxed. Allow your breath to flow smoothly and evenly. Position the band around your middle ribs, directly beneath the breast bone.
2. Now breathe in as you did for the 3D breathing exercise on page 131, and feel the resistance of the band. Fill your lungs so that your ribs expand forwards, sideways and backwards against the band. Notice if there are any differences between your left and right side. Do both sides move equally well? Can you stretch the resistance band just as much in all directions? Take 10 to 15 deep, full breaths in and out. Try not to breathe in too quickly, instead increasing the tension gradually throughout the breath. You can repeat this exercise two or three times.

› **3D breathing with respiratory training devices**

Equipment: Relaxator respiratory training device

Another way to strengthen the respiratory muscles is to use special respiratory training devices. We will be showing you a variety of equipment that can assist you with training your respiratory muscles. To create resistance for the 3D breathing exercise, we would recommend that you start with a device called a Relaxator. Later on, as you gain more experience, you can move on to using the Expand-A-Lung respiratory training device. You can find more information about these devices in the exercises on pages 140 and 149. Both respiratory training devices work by providing resistance as you inhale and exhale, which forces your respiratory muscles to work significantly harder. You can of course use any other respiratory training device that works by creating resistance as you breathe.

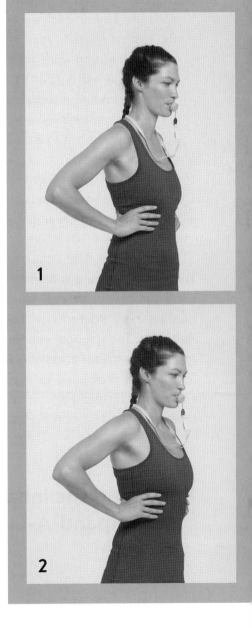

Both of the devices we recommend allow you to adjust the resistance easily and conveniently. For the following exercises, we will describe how to train using the Relaxator. The advantage of the Relaxator is that it's a handy size and doesn't weigh very much.

1. Stand with your feet hip-width apart. Lengthen your spine but keep it nice and relaxed. Allow your breath to flow smoothly and evenly. Place the Relaxator between your lips and rest your hands on either side

of your rib cage so that your thumbs are pointing backwards and your other four fingers are flat against the front of your rib cage.

2. With the resistance provided by the Relaxator, take 10 to 15 breaths in through your mouth and then breathe slowly and calmly out through your nose. Try not to breathe in too quickly. At first, increase the tension gradually as you inhale and then, as you reach the end, make your inhalations deeper and more powerful. Notice whether your fingers expand forwards, sideways and backwards as you inhale. Try to work out if there are any differences between your right and left hand. Are there parts that only move a little or not at all? If so, these sections are not fully integrated into the breathing process. The next step focuses on increasing the involvement of these parts of the lungs into your breathing. You can repeat this exercise two or three times per day.

Note: Start off with a low level of resistance and gradually work your way up. The resistance should be adjusted to allow you to breathe in all three directions at all times, while also keeping your spine and posture upright.

Strengthening the respiratory muscles using the Expand-A-Lung

The Expand-A-Lung is an excellent tool for increasing the intensity as you progress through your respiratory training and for strengthening your respiratory muscles in a targeted way. This device offers more intense resistance than the Relaxator. The stronger your respiratory muscles, the easier, more sustained and more efficient your breathing. Therefore, as well as controlling your breathing and focusing on prolonged exhalation, the strengthening of these specific muscles should be an integral element of your respiratory training. In order to target these muscles, we will be working on inhalation and exhalation as two separate systems.

❯ Training the inhalation muscles using the Expand-A-Lung

Sit or stand in a comfortable position. Lengthen your spine but keep it nice and relaxed. Choose a level of resistance that you can manage well. Place the mouthpiece of the Expand-A-Lung between your teeth and hold it gently in place with your lips. Start the respiratory training by breathing in slowly for 1 to 2 seconds and then quickly and intensely for 1 to 2 seconds, counteracting the resistance of the device. Then exhale smoothly and evenly through your nose before taking your next breath in. Make sure that your inhalation lasts no longer than 2 to 4 seconds and that your spine remains lengthened and upright. Do this breathing exercise twice a day for 10 to 15 consecutive breaths. Once you are a little more practised, increase the resistance so that the workout becomes quite strenuous after 10 to 15 repetitions.

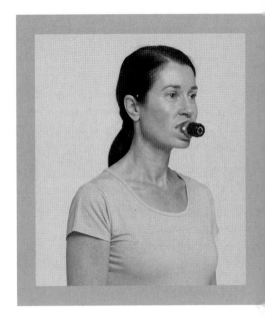

Note: It is really important to build up the tension of the inhalation slowly for about 1 to 2 seconds as described, and then inhale quickly and intensely for another 1 to 2 seconds.

› Training the exhalation muscles using the Expand-A-Lung

Sit or stand in a comfortable position. Lengthen your spine but keep it nice and relaxed. Choose a level of resistance that you find quite easy to control. Place the mouthpiece of the Expand-A-Lung between your teeth and hold it gently in place with your lips. Breathe in through your nose for 2 to 3 seconds and then control your breath as you push against the resistance to breathe out. Adjust the resistance so that one full exhalation takes 3 to 4 seconds. As you breathe, make sure that your spine stays lengthened and upright. Do this exercise twice a day with 10 to 15 breaths. Once you have got the hang of it, increase the resistance. Always select a level of intensity that makes the exercise feel strenuous after 10 to 15 breaths, but still allows you to control your posture well and keep your spine lengthened and upright.

Categorising the exercises for strengthening the respiratory muscles			
Exercise	Positive	Neutral/moderately positive	Save for later
3D breathing with a resistance band (page 138)			
3D breathing with respiratory training devices (pages 139–140)			
Relaxator			
Expand-A-Lung			
Strengthening the respiratory muscles using the Expand-A-Lung (pages 141–142)			
Training the inhalation muscles using the Expand-A-Lung (page 140)			
Training the exhalation muscles using the Expand-A-Lung (page 141)			

Training recommendations for respiratory muscle coordination

If you want to make lasting and progressive improvements to your breathing, you should start your respiratory training by improving your respiratory system mechanics in order to optimise the fundamental apparatus that controls your respiratory movements. We take a huge number of breaths each day – somewhere between 18,000 and 20,000 – all performed autonomously. If we want to make long-term changes to our breathing technique, we therefore have to counter those breaths with a vast number of optimised breaths that will have a significant effect on our nervous system. You should therefore continue this training for three to four weeks before switching to other areas.

Warm-up for respiratory training

As with the other elements involved in improving interoceptive awareness, there are some very simple and effective ways to boost our respiratory training by warming up and pre-activating our nervous system. We specifically recommend using the vagus nerve mobilisation exercises (pages 102–103) and sensory stimulus of the auricular branch exercises (pages 107–109) to activate the vagus nerve. Sensory stimulus of the auricular branch is definitely the easiest, most efficient and fastest way to prepare yourself for all aspects of your respiratory training. For this purpose, vibrating the ear for 20 to 30 seconds is sufficient.

Other useful warm-up exercises include activating the supplementary motor areas with vibrating the front teeth (page 110), bilateral wrist rotations (pages 112–113) or tongue circles (page 191). Do these exercises for 20 to 30 seconds to get the best results from your respiratory training. Make sure to use variations of the exercises for which you had positive assessment results. This will significantly increase the effectiveness and overall benefit of the training.

Improving your respiratory system mechanics as the main element of your training

As well as the exercises for coordinating the respiratory muscles, which you will have become familiar with on pages 123 to 141, improving your respiratory system mechanics also involves strengthening the respiratory muscles (pages 137–140). Both of these aspects combined will give you a good basis for further respiratory training, while also helping you to make significant improvements to your awareness of your own breathing and your breath control. The mechanical components of the breathing process activate the posterior section of the insular cortex in particular, and are therefore ideal for improving your overall interoceptive awareness. 3D breathing (page 131) works very well as part of a training plan to alleviate pelvic floor problems, while the diaphragm stretch (pages 123–124) is particularly effective for improving digestive disorders. Exercises that focus on the mechanical aspects of breathing can be done as standalone training sessions over the course of three to four weeks. Use exercises from the 'positive' or 'neutral' category. You should try to train for at least 10 to 15 minutes each day. Feel free to spread this across two or three sessions over the course of the day.

Generally speaking, the better each component of your respiratory system works, the easier and more efficient your breathing will be. The important thing here is to strengthen the muscular system that controls your breathing. Strengthening exercises for your respiratory muscles should be done three to four times a week, just like any other fitness and strength training. To do this, take 10 to 15 deep breaths two or three times consecutively, while applying resistance. The exercises are particularly effective at activating the posterior section of your insular cortex, helping to alleviate problems with digestion and the pelvic floor.

Respiratory system mechanics exercises as a warm-up for other training

The exercises designed to improve your respiratory system mechanics also make an excellent warm-up for advanced respiratory training such as prolonged exhalation or air hunger drills. 1 to 2 minutes of respiratory system mechanics exercises from the 'positive' category are all it takes to ensure a very good foundation for further training. Exercises aimed at other aspects of interoceptive awareness also benefit from a quick warm-up of your respiratory muscles. They are particularly good for helping you get the most out of your tongue training (page 186 onwards) and your pelvic floor training (page 123 onwards).

Training recommendations for respiratory muscle coordination		
Potential use	Scope and application	Effect
As a main training exercise	**Warm-up** • 20 to 30 seconds • One of the following exercises with a positive assessment result: • mobilising the vagus nerve (pages 102–103) • sensory stimulus of the auricular branch (page 107) • vibrating the front teeth (page 110) • alternating between opening and closing the hands (page 111)	• Activates the posterior section of the insular cortex • Improves: • interoceptive awareness • digestive disorders (particularly the diaphragm stretch on pages 123–124) • pelvic floor issues (particularly the 3D breathing exercises on page 131)

Training recommendations for respiratory muscle coordination		
Potential use	**Scope and application**	**Effect**
	• bilateral wrist rotations (pages 112–113) • tongue circles (page 191) **Main section** • Exercises with a positive or neutral assessment result • 10 to 15 minutes each day **Extra** • 2 to 3 rounds • 10 to 15 breaths each using the Expand-A-Lung to strengthen the respiratory muscles Carried out over the course of 3 to 4 weeks	
As a warm-up for other breathing exercises	• Exercises with positive assessment results • 1 to 2 minutes	• Activates the posterior section of the insular cortex • Improves your respiratory system mechanics for the following breathing exercises and makes the overall training more effective

As a warm-up for other interoceptive awareness exercises	• Exercises with positive assessment results
	• 1 to 2 minutes
		• Activates the posterior section of the insular cortex
		• Improves the overall effectiveness of the training
		• Particularly suitable as preparation for:
		  • pelvic floor training
		  • tongue exercises

Breathing techniques to prolong exhalation

Prolonged exhalation is, without doubt, the easiest way to alleviate many of the effects of stress on your breathing. It has a significant impact on your parasympathetic system, stimulating the vagus nerve and activating the anterior and posterior sections of your insular cortex. As well as improving your general interoceptive awareness, prolonged exhalation works brilliantly in helping to reduce chronic pain. The breath control exercises in particular, which require increased focus and attention, also activate the anterior section of the insular cortex and help to improve how we regulate emotions and feelings of anxiety. In the following section, we will first show you some simple breath control exercises to improve your awareness of your breathing and get you ready for prolonged exhalation. We will then show you a few prolonged exhalation techniques that are very efficient and are easy to fit into your daily routine.

Be aware of your breathing

As you work through the respiratory training, it's especially important that you pay full attention to your breathing at all times. The more focused and relaxed you are during the breathing exercise, as you observe the internal processes such as the movement and flow of your breath, the more effective the training will be. Focusing your attention and increasing your mindfulness as you work on your breathing can be amazingly helpful for your interoception.

❯ 4:4 breath control

The focus of this breath control exercise is initially on noticing and controlling your breathing by setting a time frame for inhalation and exhalation. Breath control with an inhalation/exhalation ratio of 4:4 is an excellent starting point for your training. Count up to four as you breathe in, and again as you breathe out. Make sure you keep the same rhythm as you count. It may help to use the second hand on a clock. You can do this exercise while walking, resting, or while doing almost any other activity. If you want to practise breath control while walking, for example, try using your walking pace to help you count. So you would inhale for four steps, then exhale for four steps. The important thing is that you breathe in through your nose evenly, keeping the breath smooth and controlled. You can choose whether to breathe out through your mouth or your nose. Exhaling through your nose makes the exercise slightly more challenging. If you have already practised positioning your tongue correctly (pages 190–191), then feel free to put your tongue in the right position during the exercise. You may find this exercise a little difficult at first, and it might make you feel short of breath. This is completely normal and nothing for you to worry about. Feel free to take a short break at any time, and just continue the exercise once you're ready. The training should last 5 to 10 minutes in total and can be carried out either once or twice a day.

Note: Once you're a little more confident with this breath control exercise, you can also add in a little pause during which you hold your breath for another 4 seconds after exhaling. So, you would breathe at an inhalation/exhalation/pause ratio of 4:4:4. This add-on requires even more control over your breathing rhythm. It also helps to normalise your blood gases and can noticeably reduce your stress levels.

❯ Variation: 2:4, 2:6 and 2:8 breath control

For these variations, you adjust the ratio of inhalation to exhalation so that you breathe out for longer than you breathe in for. Most people with increased stress levels find it difficult to exhale for longer than they inhale. That's why it's very useful to gradually increase the ratio of exhalation to inhalation. Start your breath control with a ratio of 2:4, breathing in for two counts and out for four. Once you feel comfortable with that, take the inhalation/exhalation ratio up a notch to 2:6 and then 2:8, and so on.

In practice, we often find that it's easier to start by increasing the number of counts for inhaling and exhaling, but to keep the ratio the same. So, you could start by trying a ratio of 4:8, breathing in for 4 seconds and out for 8. Feel free to play around with the different variations and use the assessments to find the ratio and number of counts that work for you. Especially when using this breathing technique while walking, we recommend choosing a higher number of counts, such as 4:8.

Prolonged exhalation using respiratory training devices

Experience shows that respiratory training equipment that requires you to exhale against an increased level of resistance is extremely effective. Firstly, breathing against resistance increases the strength and stamina of the respiratory muscles, as you have seen on pages 137 to 141. Secondly, the resistance forces you to prolong your exhalation. This reduces the effects that stress has on your breathing, which in turn has a positive effect on your blood gases, your pH value and your stress levels.

Training with a respiratory training device can easily be integrated into your daily routine. If you keep the device where you are likely to notice it as you go about your day-to-day tasks, just seeing it will prompt you to use it. In addition, it's easy to use and therefore immediately accessible to both beginners and advanced users. In this book, we use three different types of respiratory training equipment. The following exercises use the Relaxator and the Frolov respiratory training device.

❯ Prolonged exhalation using the Relaxator

The Relaxator is a simple and practical respiratory training device that enables you to do your breathing exercises any time and anywhere, with very little effort required. It also works brilliantly for achieving prolonged exhalation. To use it, inhale normally through your nose and then exhale through the Relaxator. Its handy size and the fact that it's so light means you can simply hold the Relaxator between your lips. However, it still provides you with the security and stability required to help you feel nice and relaxed while you do your respiratory training. By lightly regulating the air resistance, you can quickly adjust the intensity and exhalation time to a level that suits you.

Stand or sit in a comfortable position. Lengthen your spine but keep it nice and relaxed. Allow your breath to flow smoothly and evenly. Select a resistance level that you feel comfortable with. Place the mouthpiece between your lips and start breathing in through your nose and out through your mouth and into the Relaxator. Your jaw should be loose and relaxed. Use the Relaxator for 20 minutes a day. Feel free to use it during simple everyday activities or during a walk.

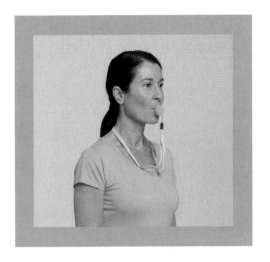

Prolonged exhalation using the Frolov respiratory training device

The Frolov respiratory trainer is another fun and easy-to-use tool for increasing awareness of and control over your breathing and making prolonged exhalation more effective. The special way in which this device works allows you to significantly lower your breathing rate during training and to significantly prolong and improve your exhalation. It works in a similar way to the Relaxator, in that you inhale through your nose and exhale into the water through the mouthpiece and the tube. If you're already quite experienced, you can try breathing in as well as out through the water in the cup. As well as assisting with prolonged exhalation, the Frolov respiratory trainer is a fun way to increase your control and tolerance of the sensation of being short of breath (page 154 onwards).

Another benefit of the Frolov respiratory trainer is that it's specially designed to provide you with complete awareness of your breathing. This allows you to control your breath and let it flow evenly. If your breathing respiratory drive becomes too strong, too sudden or too intense, you get direct feedback through the reaction of the water, which will become turbulent and splash. The water should be bubbling evenly and constantly throughout the exercise, which requires a high degree of breath control.

❯ Prolonged exhalation using the Frolov respiratory training device

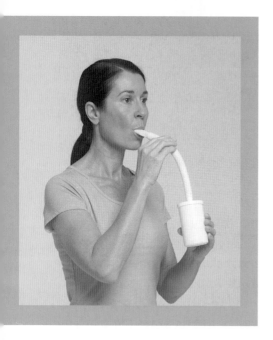

Follow the manufacturer's instructions to fill the Frolov with water. Sit or stand in a comfortable position. Lengthen your spine but keep it nice and relaxed. Hold the device in your hand and place the mouthpiece between your lips. Start by inhaling through your nose and then exhaling through the device, keeping your breath slow and controlled. Make sure that your breathing is even and controlled, sending a smooth and even jet of bubbles into the water. When you start, feel free to adjust the water level to a quantity that works best for you. The more water you use, the easier you will find it to control your breathing. Carry out the exercise with the Frolov device for 10 to 30 minutes at a time. When you first start practising, feel free to take little breaks throughout if necessary.

Note: At the beginning, you can divide your respiratory training into smaller sessions spread throughout the day, as long as you achieve a total training time of 10 to 30 minutes.

❯ Variation: Prolonged inhalation and exhalation using the Frolov respiratory training device

For this variation, do the exercise as described above, but this time breathe in through the Frolov device too. You will therefore be breathing through the resistance of the water as you inhale, as well as when you exhale. With this variation, make sure that the water level – and therefore the level of resistance – doesn't induce a feeling of breathlessness that is too far out of your comfort zone. When you first start practising, feel free to take little breaks throughout if necessary.

Note: At the beginning, you can divide your respiratory training into smaller sessions spread throughout the day, as long as you achieve a total training time of 10 to 30 minutes.

Categorising the prolonged exhalation exercises			
Exercise	Positive	Neutral/moderately positive	Save for later
4:4 breath control (pages 146–147)			
Breath control in various breathing rhythms (pages 147–148)			
2:4 breath control			
2:6 breath control			
2:8 breath control			
Prolonged exhalation using respiratory training devices			
Prolonged exhalation using the Relaxator (pages 148–149)			
Prolonged exhalation using the Frolov respiratory training device (page 150)			
Variation: Prolonged inhalation and exhalation using the Frolov respiratory training device (page 150)			

Training recommendations for prolonged exhalation

Prolonged exhalation is, without doubt, one of the most important aspects of the training, because it works so well for reducing stress, activating the vagus nerve and insular cortex, as well as for improving our general interoceptive awareness, our wellbeing and our fitness. Prolonging your exhalation has a powerful effect on your parasympathetic nervous system, helping to achieve balance and regulate stress. Practising prolonged exhalation activates the posterior and, depending on the exercise, the anterior section of your insular cortex. All exercises that require increased focus and attention, such as the breath control exercises, have a significant effect on the anterior section of the insular cortex. As a result, these exercises go a long way towards improving how we regulate emotions, as well as alleviating anxiety and depressive moods. Prolonged exhalation using the Relaxator (pages 148–149) has an especially powerful effect on the parasympathetic nervous system, and works particularly well for symptoms of anxiety. Prolonged exhalation using the Frolov respiratory training device (pages 149–150), on the other hand, is extremely effective at helping you to regulate any digestive disorders and improving your general health and stress levels.

If you're very busy and don't have much time to spare, we recommend that you integrate your respiratory training into your day-to-day life. By combining the majority of your respiratory training into your daily routine, you can do it without having to invest too much effort or additional time. It can also be really helpful to use breathing exercises as a pre-emptive measure for situations that are likely to cause stress. As mentioned at the start, we would advise doing a quick warm-up (page 144) before prolonged exhalation. Feel free to pad out the warm-up with two or three rounds of diaphragm stretches (pages 123–127). Pick one variation for which you had a positive assessment result. You should then spend at least 20 minutes on the actual prolonged exhalation exercises. You can also split this into two or three smaller sessions over the course of the day. When it comes to choosing which exercises to do, using training devices is definitely the easiest way to achieve the objectives of your respiratory training. However, you can use any exercise from the prolonged exhalation section for which you had a positive assessment and which you find comfortable to do.

Training recommendations for prolonged exhalation		
Potential use	**Scope and application**	**Effect**

As the main element of the training	**Warm-up**
	20 to 30 seconds of one of the following exercises with a positive assessment result:
	• Mobilising the vagus nerve (pages 102–103)
	• Sensory stimulus of the auricular branch (page 107)
	• Vibrating the front teeth (page 110)
	• Alternating between opening and closing the hands (page 111)
	• Bilateral wrist rotations (pages 112–113)
	• Tongue circles (page 191)
	• 2 to 3 rounds of diaphragm stretches (pages 123–124)
	
	Main section
	• Exercises with a positive or neutral assessment result
	• At least 20 minutes per day
	• Can be divided into 2 or 3 sessions
	• Feel free to use respiratory training devices
	Carried out over the course of 3 to 4 weeks
		• Activates the posterior and anterior sections of the insular cortex
		• Has a significant impact on the parasympathetic system
		• Improves:
		  • interoceptive awareness
		  • chronic pain
		  • symptoms of stress
		  • anxiety
		  • depressive moods
		  • emotional regulation

Training recommendations for prolonged exhalation		
Potential use	Scope and application	Effect
As a warm-up for other interoceptive awareness exercises	• 1 to 2 minutes • Exercises with positive assessment results	• Activates the posterior and anterior sections of the insular cortex • Improves the overall effectiveness of the training

Air hunger drills

When you look at the effects of stress on the body, breathing is almost always affected. When you are stressed, your breaths becomes shallower, shorter and quicker. In turn, this not only worsens your respiratory movements, but also interferes with the balance of oxygen and carbon dioxide in your blood. Shallow breathing causes you to take quicker and more frequent in-breaths and shorter out-breaths. This leads to insufficient levels of carbon dioxide (CO_2) in the blood, which has numerous consequences for your health. A reduction in CO_2 content can have a negative effect on the smooth muscles of the bronchi, intestines and bladder. Furthermore, having less CO_2 in your blood changes its pH value and reduces the amount of oxygen that can be transported to its destination in the body, because the CO_2 is required for binding the oxygen to the haemoglobin. CO_2 is also essential for expanding the blood vessels, thus ensuring the best possible blood circulation.

'Air hunger drills', i.e. exercises that make you feel short of breath, can raise the level of carbon dioxide in the blood back up. Air hunger drills are ideal for activating all sections of the insular cortex. They therefore work really well for anxiety, depressive moods and chronic pain, as well as improving your general interoceptive awareness, your wellbeing and your fitness levels. This is another area in which exercises that require a greater degree of focus and attention are more adept at activating the anterior section of the insular cortex. Furthermore, air hunger drills also activate important areas of the cerebellum, midbrain and brain stem. These areas have many important functions. Among other things, they are involved in processing vestibular information, spine and eye coordination, pain reduction and the regulation of posture and muscular tension. All of these aspects are directly or indirectly connected to the insular cortex.

The exhalation exercises that we have already covered also involve a mild form of air hunger. However, in the following section, we will show you a variety of simple and effective exercises you can use to create air hunger even more quickly and deliberately. The easiest way is simply to hold your breath as you move. Physical activity removes oxygen from the blood in your muscles and increases the level of carbon dioxide as a by-product. This accumulates in the blood and thus improves the ratio of carbon dioxide to oxygen. Try holding your breath while doing simple everyday activities like climbing the stairs, or fitness exercises like squats, or combine it with your usual walk to the coffee machine or the bus stop. Be creative and make the most of your time. You will find that it's actually really easy to build these air hunger drills into your daily routine, without having to find any extra time.

❯ Hold your breath

As described earlier, this exercise simply requires you to hold your breath while doing light or moderate physical activity. You will feel the urge to inhale very quickly. The aim is to learn to consciously control the urge to inhale, and to gradually leave it longer and longer before you do breathe in. It's also really important that you train yourself to resume a calm, balanced breathing rhythm as soon as possible after the exercise. Can you breathe normally again within two to three breaths? Try it – practice makes perfect!

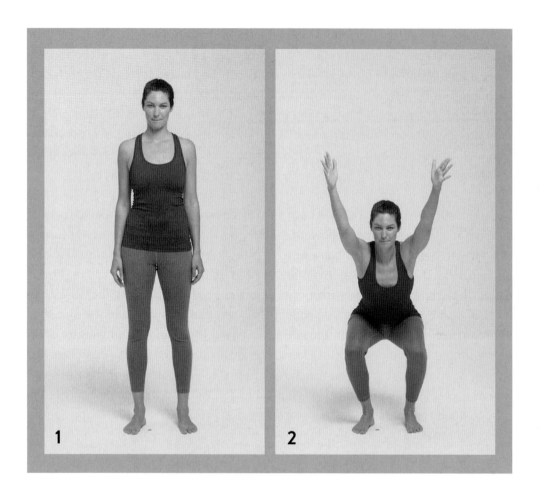

1. Stand with your feet hip to shoulder-distance apart. Lengthen your spine but keep it nice and relaxed. Close your mouth and hold your breath.
2. Start by doing a physical activity of your choice. That might be walking, a gentle jog, squats, lunges, or something similar. When you feel a strong urge to inhale, stop the movement and breathe in. Try to return to a calm and even breathing rhythm as quickly as possible. As you practise the exercise, gradually try to control the urge to inhale and delay it for longer each time. You can repeat this exercise two or three times.

❯ Variation 1: Exhale and hold your breath

A slightly harder but very effective variation is to do this exercise after breathing out. You don't need to fully exhale for this. It's fine to just exhale some of the air in your lungs before holding your breath and doing your chosen activity. This variation makes you feel much more out of breath much more quickly too, giving you a really strong urge to breathe in. The important thing is to maintain a sense of control. This exercise shouldn't make you feel excessively uncomfortable.

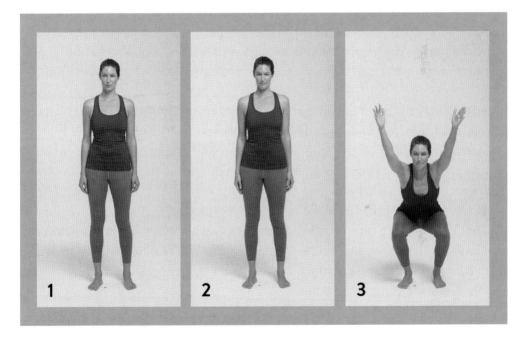

1. Stand with your feet hip to shoulder-distance apart. Lengthen your spine but keep it nice and relaxed. Exhale some of your breath through your mouth.
2. Then close your mouth and hold your breath.
3. Choose a physical activity that isn't too strenuous, such as walking, gently jogging, squats, lunges or something similar. Carry out your chosen movement while holding your breath until you feel a strong urge to inhale. Then stop what you're doing and try to resume your normal breathing rhythm – smooth and even – as quickly as possible. As you practise the exercise, gradually try to

control the urge to inhale and delay it for longer each time. You can repeat this exercise two or three times.

❯ Variation 2: Cross coordination with breath hold

The cross coordination with breath hold drill is a special variation of the standard breath hold drill. It works particularly well as warm-up for sports because it has so many positive effects on any subsequent training activity. Cross coordination improves the communication between the two halves of the brain, as well as increasing activity in both halves of the cerebellum. If you haven't yet noticed many changes as you've progressed through your training, you should find it helpful to make the air hunger drill with cross coordination part of your warm-up.

1. Stand with your feet hip-width apart. Lengthen your spine but keep it nice and relaxed. Close your mouth and hold your breath.
2. Start by marching on the spot, keeping a steady rhythm. Once you've found your rhythm, cross your right hand over to your left knee.
3. Then cross your left hand over to your right knee. As you do this, your knee and hand should cross over the centre of your body.
4. Continue crossing alternate hands and knees while holding your breath until you feel a strong urge to inhale. Then stop what you're doing and try to return to a smooth and even breathing rhythm as quickly as possible. You can repeat this exercise two or three times.

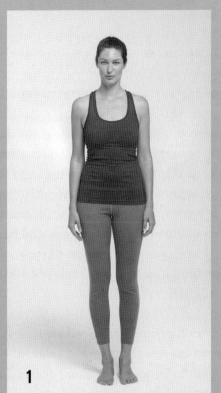

1

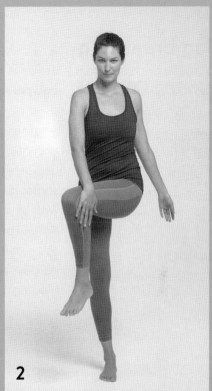

2

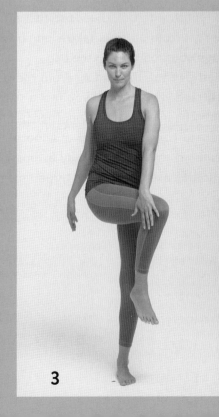

3

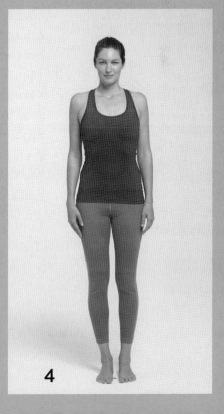

4

› Bag breathing

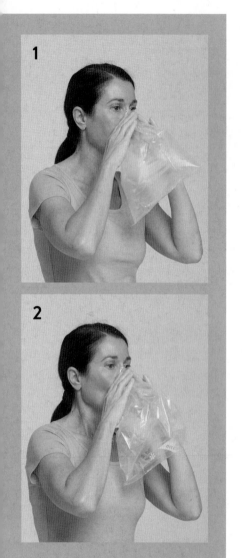

Equipment: Bag with approx. 3 litres of capacity

Another exercise that helps make up for the depletion of CO_2 caused by stress-induced breathing is bag breathing. This technique is often used when someone is hyperventilating, which can happen with severe anxiety or panic attacks, for example. When you breathe into a bag, you breathe back in the exhaled air containing carbon dioxide, which quickly compensates for any imbalance in the blood gases.

1. Sit or stand in a comfortable position. Lengthen your spine but keep it nice and relaxed. Allow your breath to flow smoothly and evenly. Take a paper or plastic bag and hold it tight over your nose and mouth with both hands so that no air can get into it from outside. Take a long breath out through your mouth into the bag.
2. Then breathe in the exhaled air from the bag. Keep breathing like this until you feel a strong urge to breathe in normally again. Then put the bag aside and try to return to a smooth and even breathing rhythm as quickly as possible. You can do this exercise two or three times in succession.

› Simplified bag breathing

Equipment: Bag with approx. 3 litres of capacity

With this simplified variation, you leave a little space between the bag and your nose and mouth. This allows you to breathe in a little fresh air with each inhalation, which lowers the intensity of the exercise and doesn't make you feel short of breath quite so quickly. This variation is ideal for people who find the exercise too uncomfortable when their mouth and nose are covered, as well as for all those who feel out of breath very quickly during the basic exercise.

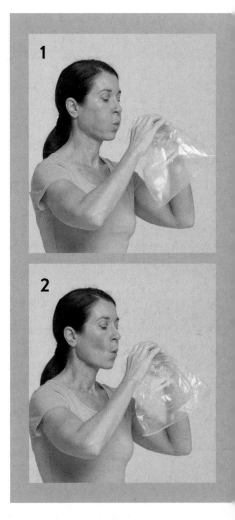

1. Sit or stand in a comfortable position. Lengthen your spine but keep it nice and relaxed. Allow your breath to flow smoothly and evenly. Take a paper or plastic bag and hold it briefly with both hands over your nose and mouth. Then move the bag 2 to 5 cm away from your face. Now take a long breath out into the bag.
2. Then breathe the exhaled air back in. Continue breathing like this until you feel a strong urge to inhale normally. Then place the bag to one side and try to return to a smooth and even breathing rhythm as quickly as possible. You can repeat this exercise two or three times.

Try to get used to the feeling of breathlessness!

At first, some people find bag breathing really strange and it may make them feel uncomfortable or anxious. However, most people get used to the exercise the more they practise. That said, make sure that you feel safe during this exercise and that you always feel in control. If bag breathing causes too much discomfort, feel free to use the other air hunger drills instead.

Categorising the air hunger drills			
Exercise	Positive	Neutral/moderately positive	Save for later
Hold your breath (pages 155–156)			
Variation 1: Exhale and hold your breath (pages 157–158)			
Variation 2: Cross coordination with breath hold (pages 158–159)			
Bag breathing (page 160)			
Simplified bag breathing (page 161)			

Training recommendations for the use of air hunger drills

Air hunger drills can be used for various different purposes. For example, they can quickly alleviate symptoms of exertion or stress. Because they activate all sections of the insular cortex, air hunger drills also help to improve our general interoceptive awareness and work well as a warm-up for further interoceptive training.

Air hunger drills for coping with stress

Bag breathing can be used as a short-term remedy to quickly alleviate symptoms of stress. However, other air hunger drills can do this too. In intensely stressful situations, carry out two to four air hunger drills in quick succession, if circumstances allow. If not, you can use slightly less conspicuous exercises such as prolonged exhalation (pages 146–149), which is a less intense variation of an air hunger drill. Do the air hunger drills five to eight times a day until you notice a reduction in your stress symptoms.

Air hunger drills as part of interoceptive awareness training

As well as providing immediate relief for symptoms of stress and anxiety, air hunger drills affect all areas of your insular cortex and are therefore very effective for alleviating chronic pain, anxiety, depressive moods and generally improving your health, wellbeing and fitness. You can also combine the air hunger drills with other elements of your interoceptive awareness, doing them in conjunction with other exercises. Try holding your breath one to three times while doing the tongue exercises (page 186 onwards), balance exercises (page 66) or pelvic floor training (page 170 onwards) before continuing with the exercise. This is comparable to the basic air hunger exercise (pages 155–156), which simply involves carrying out air hunger drills while doing everyday activities. You should try to do a daily total of at least 5 to 10 minutes of air hunger drills. Feel free to spread them out into two or three smaller sessions over the course of the day.

Air hunger drills as a warm-up for other training exercises

You can also use air hunger drills as a way of warming up for other exercises in this book. Because air hunger drills affect the central section of the insular cortex, they also improve integration and therefore are an excellent way of preparing your body to train other aspects of your interoceptive awareness. The fact that they also increase the levels of CO_2 in your blood means they have many positive physiological and neural effects. You can use these effects to get the most out of your training. To do this, choose one to three exercises for which you had a positive assessment result and carry these out for a total of 1 to 3 minutes before your main training.

Training recommendations for the use of air hunger drills		
Potential use	**Scope and application**	**Effect**
For immediate stress reduction	• 1 exercise with positive assessment result • 2 to 4 rounds • 5 to 8 times per day	Reduces stress and anxiety

Training recommendations for the use of air hunger drills		
Potential use	**Scope and application**	**Effect**

As part of interoception training	• Exercises with a positive or neutral assessment result
	• 5 to 10 minutes each day
	• Works well combined with:
	  • tongue exercises
	  • pelvic floor training
	  • vestibular training
		• Activates the posterior, central and anterior sections of the insular cortex
		• Improves:
		  • chronic pain
		  • anxiety
		  • depressive moods
		  • emotional regulation
		  • general health, fitness and wellbeing

As a warm-up for other interoceptive awareness exercises	• Exercises with positive assessment results • 1 to 2 minutes	• Activates the posterior, central and anterior sections of the insular cortex • Improves the capacity for integration • Improves the overall effectiveness of the training

How to use the respiratory training techniques

As you saw in this chapter, respiratory training covers three main areas: 'Improving the coordination of your respiratory muscles' (pages 121–145), 'Breathing techniques to prolong exhalation' (pages 146–154) and 'Air hunger drills' (pages 154–164). Try using each of these areas as the main element of your training, giving it your full attention over the course of a few weeks. Training recommendations can be found at the bottom of each section. Once you're familiar with the exercises and have got the hang of the basics, you can try combining them with other exercises to form the main part or just a small part of your interoceptive awareness training.

Combining all the elements for a comprehensive respiratory training

If you want to combine all the different breathing exercises into one long training session, we recommend the following sequence:

1. Start with a short warm-up to pre-activate the vagus nerve (page 143).
2. Then do two or three rounds of air hunger drills for which you had a positive assessment result (pages 155–161).
3. Then move to 4 or 5 minutes of exercises for improving your respiratory system mechanics (pages 123–141).
4. Follow that up with 10 to 15 breaths using a respiratory training device, to strengthen the respiratory muscles (pages 140–141).
5. Finish the session with 10 to 15 minutes of prolonged exhalation, for which you can use one technique or combine a few (pages 146–150).

By combining all the different breathing exercises, you will easily manage a total training time of 20 to 30 minutes per day. If you prefer, you can split this into two or three shorter sessions. Continue this training for between four and six weeks.

Recommendations for combining all the elements for a comprehensive respiratory training		
Potential use	**Scope and application**	**Effect**

Combining all the breathing exercises as the main element of your training	**Warm-up**
	 20 to 30 seconds of one of the following exercises with a positive assessment result:
	 • Mobilising the vagus nerve (pages 102–103)
	 • Sensory stimulus of the auricular branch (page 107)
	 • Vibrating the front teeth (page 110)
		• Activates all sections of the insular cortex
		 • Improves:
		   • interoceptive awareness
		   • general health, fitness and wellbeing
		 • stress

Continued on next page

Continued from page 165

Recommendations for combining all the elements for a comprehensive respiratory training		
Potential use	**Scope and application**	**Effect**

Combining all the breathing exercises as the main element of your training	• Alternating between opening and closing the hands (page 111)
	• Bilateral wrist rotations (pages 112–113)
	• Tongue circles (page 191)
	
	Air hunger drills
	• 1 exercise with positive assessment result
	• 2 to 3 rounds
	
	Improving the coordination of your respiratory muscles
	• Exercises with positive assessment results
	• 4 to 5 minutes
	• Plus 10 to 15 breaths each using the respiratory training device to strengthen the respiratory muscles
	
	Prolonged exhalation
	• 1 to 2 exercises with positive assessment results
	• 10 to 15 minutes
	
	Total training time
	• 20 to 30 minutes each day
	• Feel free to divide this into 2 or 3 smaller sessions
	• Carried out over the course of 4 to 6 weeks
		• Improves:
		  • physiological and neural foundations
		  • emotional regulation
		  • capacity for integration
		  • chronic pain

The pelvic floor – an essential component of interoceptive awareness

Despite often being overlooked, training the pelvic floor is an excellent way to improve interoception. We would therefore strongly recommend that you incorporate pelvic floor exercises into your training. The pelvic floor muscles are innervated through the interaction between the sympathetic and the parasympathetic nervous systems. Information generated by the movements of the pelvic floor is transmitted to the insular cortex, where it activates the posterior section. You can use this area of the insular cortex to improve various aspects of your physical health. For example, focusing on the pelvic floor has been proven to effect a significant improvement in digestive problems. In a sense, the pelvic floor is the lowest area from which interoceptive information comes. Together with the mouth and throat area, it can be said that the pelvic floor forms the upper and lower 'framework' of interoceptive awareness.

The pelvic floor has many important functions that we need to maintain and support as best we can. On the one hand, it closes the pelvis and therefore supports our internal organs. In women, this includes the uterus, which is particularly important during pregnancy. It also ensures that the sphincters of the bladder and intestines can do their jobs properly, as well as playing a part in various aspects of sexuality. Isolated pelvic floor training is often a difficult and lengthy process.

The pelvic floor consists of several layers, which have minimal representation in the brain, both in sensory and motor areas. In other words, the areas representing the pelvic floor in the brain are only very small, which makes it extremely difficult to have a good awareness of it and to be able to change the way we control it. The signals that run between the pelvic floor and the brain often aren't strong enough either, which means pelvic floor training alone is usually not sufficient to effect lasting neuroplastic change. When we focus on the neural aspects and the functional networks to which the pelvic floor belongs, pelvic floor training becomes much easier and more sustainable.

The particularities of the female pelvic floor

If we look at the size and shape of the pelvis in women, we see that it has different mechanical properties to that of men. Furthermore, the pelvic floor is placed under particular strain during pregnancy and childbirth. Often, our lifestyles do not allow for adequate rest and recovery in the postpartum period, which means that further strain is often placed on the pelvic floor in the days and weeks following delivery and the process of uterine regression is disrupted. This often leads to impairments in the health and functioning of the pelvic floor. That's why we are so keen to stress how important it is to address these problems. By preparing and activating the specific neural pathways connected with the pelvic floor, we can achieve vast improvements in this important area even years after pregnancy and childbirth.

Like most structures that are located in the core, the pelvic floor works bilaterally. This means that both sides of the pelvic floor have to be coordinated and controlled simultaneously. Therefore, working on the areas of the brain that are involved in the coordination and stability of bilateral movements is the perfect way to warm up for and support your pelvic floor training. Exercises that activate the supplementary motor areas (page 109 onwards) work particularly well here, as do tongue and breathing exercises, since these are also closely related to the pelvic floor, both functionally and through shared neural networks. The coordination and control of both sides of the diaphragm and pelvic floor is synchronised for the

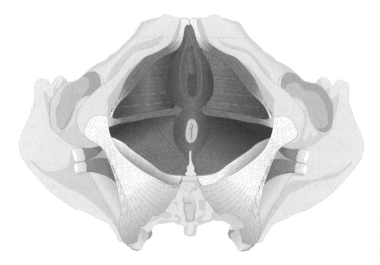

The pelvic floor muscles close the pelvis, support the organs and help to regulate the excretory system.

most part, with each side working together as one unit. Further instructions on how to warm up for the pelvic floor exercises can be found in the training recommendations at the end of this chapter (pages 179–181). Feel free to use these as a quick warm-up to make the individual exercises easier and more effective.

In order to make the pelvic floor training easier for you, let's take a look at the structure of the pelvic floor. The pelvic floor muscles are divided into two layers: a superficial level (skin level) and a deeper level, which is around 2.5 to 3 cm further down. In simple terms, there are two different lines of muscle in the pelvic floor, one of which runs transversely across the body from one sit bone to the other, while the other runs lengthways from the tailbone to the pubic bone. The path of the muscles is used in the following to describe the directions of the muscle contractions and to give you a good visual representation to help guide you.

Use the cross in the illustration opposite as a guide. The lines of the cross represent the transverse connection of the sit bones and the lengthways connection from the pubic bone to the tailbone. You can contract each different layer from the outside inwards. To do this, you either start from the right and left sit bones, or from the pubic bone at the front and the tailbone at the back. As you contract the muscles, all four corner points are pulled inwards, and as you release them, they relax outwards.

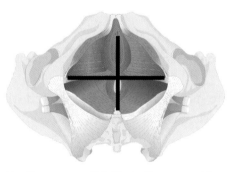

Use the cross on this illustration as a guide to help you visualise the directions in which the pelvic floor muscles contract.

Pelvic floor training can be quite difficult to start with, as most people don't know how to control this area, which is so deep inside the core. It can be helpful to visualise the pelvic floor muscles moving inside your body. Try to imagine the movement and give yourself clear instructions on how and where to move. The cross should help you to get a good idea of how the muscles move. In the following section, we will show you a series of simple and effective exercises that are easy to do even if you've never done any pelvic floor training before.

Conscious relaxation is the key to more strength and control

Although pelvic floor training is always about strengthening and improving the function of the muscles, as well as being part of our overall interoception training, we mustn't forget that most people hold too much tension in some areas of the pelvic floor. However, this does not mean that training the muscles is unnecessary. It's more a case of learning how to relax the pelvic floor again after tensing it. So, each time you actively tense the pelvic floor, make sure you give yourself enough time to relax it again. When you first start, you should spend about three to four times longer relaxing the pelvic floor than you do tensing it.

〉 Training the superficial layer: tensing the pelvic floor between the sit bones

Equipment: Mat or other comfortable surface

To make it easier to get started with pelvic floor training, you should learn the basic exercises while lying down and start by contracting your pelvic floor from the outside in. Lying down and contracting the muscles from the outside in will make it easier for you to access this area, which can be difficult to reach at first.

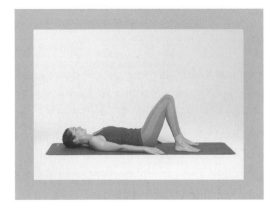

Lie on your back with your spine lengthened and relaxed, your knees bent and your feet flat on the floor. Make sure that your spine is in a natural position and that you don't put too much pressure on the hollow of your back or press your lower back against the floor. From this position, tense your pelvic floor by trying to pull the sit bones together at skin level by contracting your pelvic floor muscles. Try to ensure that you're only contracting the superficial layer of the pelvic floor and that your glutes and inner thigh muscles (adductors) stay relaxed. Hold the tension in this part of the superficial layer of your pelvic floor for 3 to 6 seconds and then relax the pelvic floor completely. This can take 10 to 20 seconds. Feel free to do the exercise between three and eight times in a row.

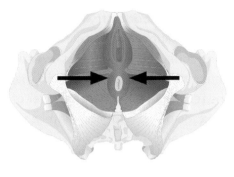

Draw both sit bones towards the middle.

❭ Training the superficial layer: tensing the pelvic floor between the pubic bone and the tailbone

Equipment: Mat or other comfortable surface

Lie on your back with your spine lengthened and relaxed, your knees bent and your feet flat on the floor. Make sure that your spine is in a natural position and that you don't put too much pressure on the hollow of your back or press your lower back too far into the floor. From this position, tense the superficial layer of

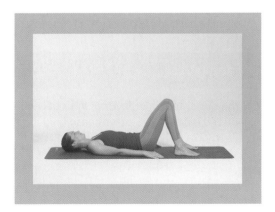

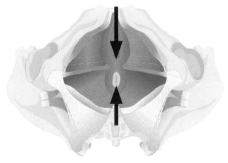

Draw the pubic bone and tailbone in towards the middle.

your pelvic floor by trying to bring the pubic bone and the tailbone together at skin level above the muscles of the pelvic floor. Try to make sure that you're only contracting the upper-most layer of the pelvic floor, at skin level. There shouldn't be any tension in your glutes or the adductors that pull your legs together. Hold the tension in the superficial layer of your pelvic floor for 3 to 6 seconds and then relax the pelvic floor completely. This can take 10 to 20 seconds. Repeat the contraction and relaxation between three and eight times.

❯ Training the superficial layer: the diamond

This exercise is a combination of the previous two. This time, rather than only contracting the muscles either transversely or lengthways, you will draw all four corners of the superficial layer of the pelvic floor towards the middle at the same time.

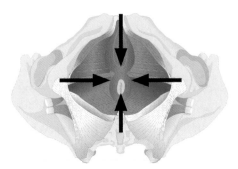

Draw both sit bones as well as the pubic bone and tailbone in towards the middle.

Relax your thighs and glutes

It will take a little time before you can control the outer and inner layer of your pelvic floor in isolation. In the beginning, the glutes and the inner thighs often tense up during pelvic floor training, which makes it difficult to precisely control the pelvic floor muscles. That's why it's so important to try to keep the glutes and inner thighs relaxed while you are doing your pelvic floor exercises.

❯ Training the deep layer: tensing the pelvic floor between the sit bones

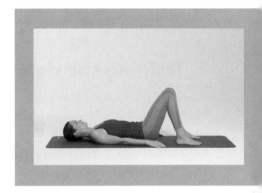

Lie on your back with your spine lengthened and relaxed, your knees bent and your feet flat on the floor. Make sure that your spine is in a natural position and that you don't put too much pressure on the hollow of your back or press your lower back into the floor. From this position, tense your pelvic floor, using the deeper muscles that lie around 3 cm down to pull your sit bones together and your pelvic floor inwards and upwards. The crucial thing is that the contraction comes from the deeper layer of the pelvic floor. Hold the tension in the deep layer of your pelvic floor for 3 to 6 seconds and then relax your pelvic floor completely. This can take 10 to 20 seconds. It's often really difficult to locate and contract the deeper layer at first. Just remember, there's no rush!

❯ Training the deep layer: tensing the pelvic floor between the pubic bone and the tailbone

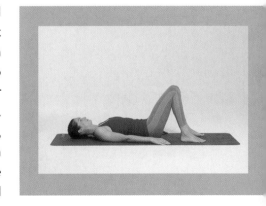

Lie on your back with your spine lengthened and relaxed, your knees bent and your feet flat on the floor. Make sure that your spine is in a natural position and that you don't put too much pressure on the hollow of your back or press your lower back too far into the floor. From this position, tense your pelvic floor, using the deeper muscles that lie around 3 cm down to pull your tailbone and pubic bone together and your pelvic floor inwards and upwards. Hold the tension in the deep layer of your pelvic floor for 3 to 6 seconds and then relax your pelvic floor completely. This can take 10 to 20 seconds. It's often really difficult to locate and contract the deeper layer at first. Take your time – there's no rush!

❯ Training the deep layer: the diamond

In the deep layer, too, you should work towards contracting the muscles in both directions simultaneously, drawing both sit bones and your tailbone and pubic bone into the middle at once. Again, this exercise is a combination of the previous two. Bring all four corners of the pelvic floor into the middle at once.

❯ Tensing and relaxing the whole pelvic floor

Once you have got the hang of tensing and relaxing the upper and lower layers of your pelvic floor separately, you can try to exercise both layers at the same time. The next step is therefore to tense your entire pelvic floor. This exercise requires an even greater awareness of what's happening in your core. You should only attempt it once you've mastered the basic exercises.

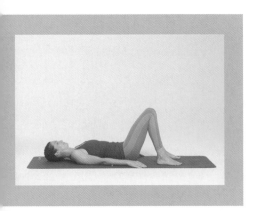

Lie on your back, with your spine lengthened and relaxed, your knees bent and your feet flat on the floor. From this position, start by tensing the outer and upper layer and then the lower layer of your pelvic floor in both directions at the same time for 3 to 5 seconds. Then relax it completely. Do you feel the same degree of contraction in both layers? Do both layers relax equally or does one layer take a little more time? Explore these questions and try to notice these important differences.

❯ Differentiating the pelvic floor muscles

As we mentioned in the basic exercises, training just the pelvic floor is difficult, as you have to prevent your glutes and adductors from tensing up at the same time. The reverse is also true, in that your pelvic floor is often much too active and tenses when you use your glutes or adductors. The next exercise therefore aims to improve your ability to differentiate and isolate the pelvic floor muscles from the glutes and adductors. First you will tense the pelvic floor and glutes, then you will relax just the pelvic floor, so that only the glutes remain tense. Before you attempt this advanced exercise, you need to have had plenty of practice with the basic exercises and to be comfortable relaxing the pelvic floor properly. The exercise calls for a significant capacity for differentiation, and therefore has a particularly powerful effect on the insular cortex.

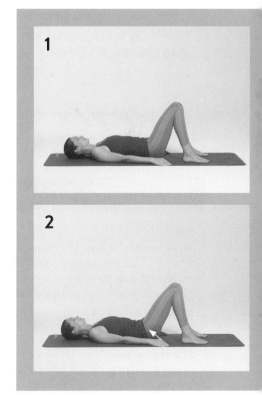

1. Lie on your back, with your spine lengthened and relaxed, your knees bent and your feet flat on the floor. Make sure that your spine is in a neutral position and that you don't put too much pressure on the hollow of your back or press your lower back too far into the floor.
2. From this position, contract both layers of the pelvic floor, while also tensing your glutes by squeezing your buttocks together. Hold this tension for 5 to 10 seconds and then slowly relax your pelvic floor while maintaining the contraction in your glutes. Once your pelvic floor is completely relaxed, slowly release the tension in your glutes. Repeat this exercise three or four times.

Note: Remember that relaxing the pelvic floor takes time. Give yourself plenty of time to learn this exercise and practise it regularly until you are really confident making the important distinction between the pelvic floor and the surrounding muscles.

❭ Variation: Pelvic floor exercises in a step position

We will now show you a series of pelvic floor exercises that you can do with one foot in front of the other. This is one example of the different ways in which you can train yourself to tense and relax the pelvic floor and glutes either simultaneously or in isolation.

1. Stand with one foot in front of the other. Your feet should not be too far apart – make sure that both heels are firmly on the floor and your legs are straight, with the centre of gravity in the middle, so that your weight is evenly distributed across both feet. Lengthen your spine but keep it nice and relaxed. Allow your breath to flow smoothly and evenly.

2. Start by contracting both layers of the pelvic floor and your glutes. Hold this tension for 5 to 10 seconds and then relax just your pelvic floor, keeping your glutes contracted. Once your pelvic floor is completely relaxed, release the tension in your glutes. Then switch the position of your legs so that your other foot is in front this time, and repeat the contraction and relaxation. Do this exercise three or four times.

Note: This exercise is very advanced and requires you to have an excellent awareness of your body.

Pelvic floor exercises in different positions

There are several ways to make your pelvic floor training more interesting and to add some variety to the exercises, giving you even more control over the tension and relaxation and building in new and different positions and movements. For example, you can try starting from a deep crouch or lunge position. Adapting the exercise to various different poses and scenarios gives your pelvic floor the best possible preparation for everyday demands.

If you learned the basic exercises and how to differentiate the pelvic floor muscles while lying down, you should also have a go at doing them in specific poses and positions. You can perform all of the exercises while sitting, standing, crouching deeply, lunging or even in different yoga poses. Feel free to get creative! The only essential thing is to try different positions that cover a wide range of movements.

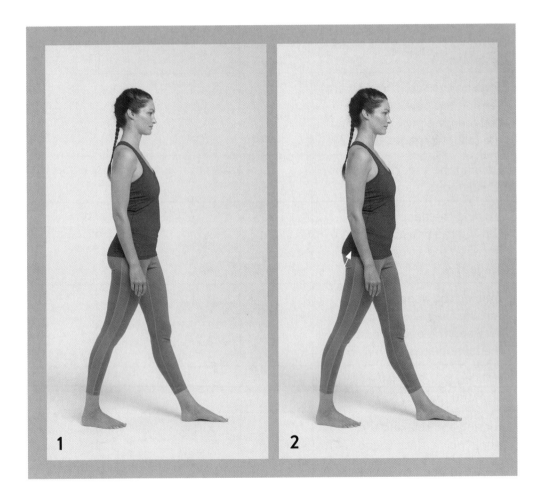

Categorising the pelvic floor exercises			
Exercise	Positive	Neutral/moderately positive	Save for later
Training the superficial layer: Tensing the pelvic floor between the sit bones (pages 170–171)			
Training the superficial layer: Tensing the pelvic floor between the pubic bone and the tailbone (pages 171–172)			
Training the superficial layer: the diamond (page 172)			
Training the deep layer: Tensing the pelvic floor between the sit bones (page 173)			
Training the deep layer: Tensing the pelvic floor between the pubic bone and the tailbone (pages 173–174)			
Training the deep layer: the diamond (page 174)			
Tensing and relaxing the whole pelvic floor (page 174)			
Differentiating the pelvic floor muscles (page 175)			
Variation: Pelvic floor exercises in a step position (pages 176–177)			

Recommendations for pelvic floor training

While the basic pelvic floor exercises mainly activate the posterior section of the insular cortex, the different positions and the differentiation exercises also activate the anterior section. This makes them ideal for improving our emotional regulation, our general interoceptive awareness, our health and wellbeing, as well as for reducing stress. The basic exercises, on the other hand, have positive effects on digestive problems and – due to the mechanical conditions – help to alleviate pain, especially in the core. Of course, all the exercises also improve pelvic floor problems.

As we mentioned in the introduction (page 168), the key to successful pelvic floor training is to warm up your system by activating the supplementary motor areas. This improves your ability to coordinate and control the different muscles. Combining vibrating the front teeth (page 110) with synchronised coordination of your hand movements works particularly well, using the exercises 'alternating between opening and closing the hands' (page 111) and 'bilateral wrist rotations' (pages 112–113). As with the respiratory training, you can also achieve great results with the tongue exercises from Chapter 5 (pages 186–199) and activating the throat area by 'gargling' (pages 205–206) and 'swallowing' (pages 207–208). We would like to reiterate that, because the pelvic floor is often so difficult to train, you should make use of all the neural activation and preparation exercises available to you in order to make your training easier and achieve more lasting effects.

Because breathing and the pelvic floor are so closely related to each other – both neurally and functionally – you should do your pelvic floor training either just after your respiratory training or following a short 1–2 minute breathing exercise of your choice. The 3D breathing exercise on page 131 works particularly well for this.

Pelvic floor exercises as the main element of your training

To achieve the improvements and results you want, we recommend that you start by making pelvic floor exercises the main element of your training. Only when you have a really good grasp of the pelvic floor exercises should you use them as a way to improve your general interoceptive awareness. To do this, try combining individual exercises for which you have achieved positive assessment results with exercises from other areas of interoceptive awareness to obtain a broad range of interoceptive information. We will show you how to do this in the next section. You should warm up your body for pelvic floor training by doing 2 to 5 minutes of breathing exercises and activating the supplementary motor areas. You should then go on to train for about 10 minutes, at least once a day. When you first start, limit yourself to the basic exercises and follow the order specified in this book. It can take several weeks to see significant improvement.

If you are really adept at the pelvic floor exercises, you should move on to the advanced exercises that involve differentiating the muscles and building in different positions (pages 175–177). Start with the recommended sequence of exercises here, too. Once you have mastered the more challenging exercises, you can switch back and forth between the exercises as you wish. However, we always recommend that you repeat the basic exercises regularly.

Pelvic floor exercises as part of interoceptive awareness training

To use the pelvic floor exercises to increase your general interoceptive awareness, the best approach is to incorporate the pelvic floor exercises into your training for 3 to 4 minutes after doing a series of tongue or breathing exercises. We would advise that you only use one aspect of the pelvic floor training and change it about once a week. This way, you always have enough time to improve these specific areas, which are otherwise quite difficult to train.

Recommendations for pelvic floor training		
Potential use	**Scope and application**	**Effect**

As the main element of the training	**Warm-up**
	1 to 2 minutes of one of the following exercises with positive assessment results:
	• Vibrating the front teeth (page 110)
	• Alternating between opening and closing the hands (page 111)
	• Bilateral wrist rotations (pages 112–113)
	• Tongue exercises (pages 186–199)
	• Activating the throat area (pages 204–208)
	• 3D breathing (page 131)
	
	Main training
	• Exercises with a positive or neutral assessment result
	• Starting with the basic exercises
	• 10 to 15 minutes
	• 1 to 2 times per day
	• Carried out over the course of 4 to 6 weeks
		Basic exercises
		• Activate the posterior section of the insular cortex
		• Improves:
		  • pelvic floor problems
		  • digestive problems
		  • pain symptoms, especially pain in the core
		
		Differentiating the pelvic floor muscles (page 175) and variation of the pelvic floor exercise with one foot in front of the other (pages 176–177)
		• Activate the posterior and anterior sections of the insular cortex
		• Improves:
		  • interoceptive awareness
		  • stress
		  • health and general wellbeing
		  • emotional regulation

As part of interoceptive awareness training	• Exercises with positive assessment results • 1 to 2 minutes • Do this 2 to 3 times per day	

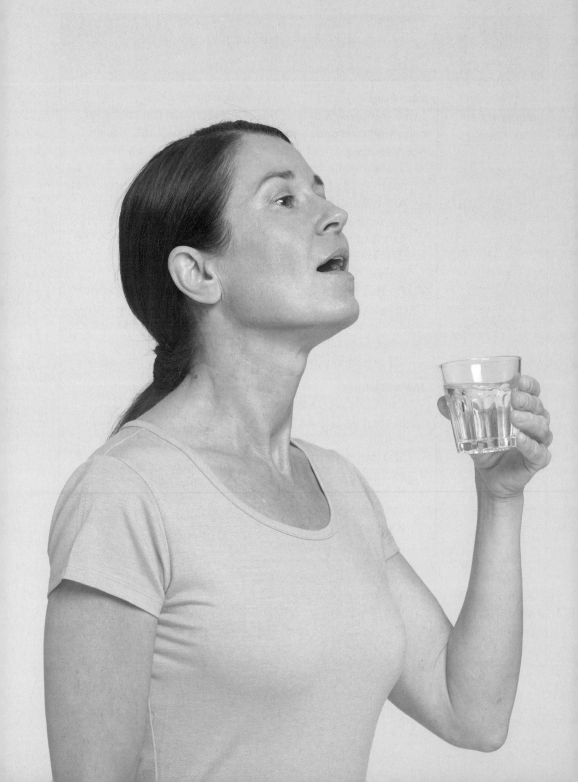

5

Tongue and throat

Impacting the vagus nerve and interoceptive awareness with tongue exercises

Most people are unaware of how important the tongue is for the functionality of the brain and nervous system. Its potential for improving our general health is therefore often overlooked. If you take a closer look at what the tongue actually does, you can clearly see that it plays an important role in our interoceptive awareness. Among other things, it is involved in breathing, eating, speaking, facial expressions and stabilising the jaw, head and neck. From a neurocentric approach, therefore, the influence of the tongue is enormous.

All parts of the body are represented in a corresponding area of the brain. In simple terms, this is where the information from these parts of the body is processed. Many large areas are assigned to the tongue and the oral cavity. The information received about the movement and feeling of the tongue is able to generate a lot of activity in the areas of the brain that represent it, thus activating large parts of the whole brain. The receptors responsible for perceiving tastes are also on the tongue. This particular area is so important for interoceptive awareness that we have dedicated a separate section to it in Chapter 3, on pages 94 to 97.

Furthermore, the tongue is innervated by several major cranial nerves that affect the regulation of autonomous functions. This includes the vagus nerve. As well as the impact of the signals that are transmitted directly to the insular cortex via the vagus nerve, there are many other ways in which tongue exercises can improve interoceptive awareness. First of all, the tongue is an organ located inside the body. This means the information received from this area is interoceptive by its very nature. Tongue movements improve the activation of the supplementary motor areas (page 109), which in turn provides a good foundation for honing our interoceptive awareness. Another important factor that makes tongue exercises so effective is the position of the areas in the brain that represent the sensory and motor aspects of the tongue. These are located directly above and adjacent to the insular cortex. Due to the physical proximity of these parts of the brain, moving the tongue, perceiving the movements of the tongue and using the tongue to touch and feel, all lead to increased blood supply and neural activity in this area. The increased blood supply and consequent increase in neural activity also extends to the insular cortex, adjacent to the area. As well as activating the insular cortex by increasing its blood supply, the information from the tongue also travels to the posterior section of the insular cortex, leading to an increase in its activity levels. Tongue exercises are therefore extremely effective for improving predominantly physical complaints such as digestion and pelvic floor problems.

Activating the supplementary motor areas by moving the tongue has a very positive effect on pelvic floor training. In addition, tongue exercises optimise the perception and control of our eye movements and support the vestibular system. These two systems, especially the vestibular system, play a crucial role in optimising the regulation and control of internal processes (Chapter 3, pages 64–65). As well as the tongue playing a key part in our interoceptive awareness, its sensory and motor functions also activate the part of the brain stem that is heavily involved in regulating breathing, cardiac activity and muscular tension, all of which are also important aspects of interoceptive awareness. Last but not least, the powerful stimuli that are transmitted to the brain via the tongue increase the levels of neural activity in many parts of the brain. This in turn makes the brain more capable of adapting to different conditions.

The exercises for training the tongue are structured as follows: We will start with sensory exercises. The aim here is to improve the tongue's ability to perceive touch by deliberately stimulating it. This will be followed by a series of exercises designed to help coordinate and strengthen the tongue muscles. Because the tongue has a wide range of movement, we have selected exercises that cover this whole range in order to provide comprehensive training. To round off the most important aspects of your tongue training, the first part of this chapter concludes with a series of exercises designed to help you stretch the tongue muscles.

Improving the perception of the tongue with sensory stimulus

Sensory stimulation of the tongue makes the perfect warm-up for further tongue training. As you will see, preparing in this way makes the tongue movements easier and more fluid. Stimulating the tongue also helps to prepare you for throat exercises in which the tongue is also involved, such as humming, gargling and swallowing, and usually makes these exercises much easier to do.

Note for all tongue exercises

Try not to move your jaw while you're doing the tongue exercises and keep your head, neck and face as relaxed as possible.

❭ Sensory stimulation of the tongue using the Z-Vibe

Equipment: Z-Vibe or electric toothbrush

Probably the easiest and quickest way to trigger a large quantity of sensory information via the tongue is by using the Z-Vibe, which we introduced in Chapter 3 on page 107. This device, which was specially developed for use in the oral cavity, has different surface structures that enable you to train and activate the tongue's

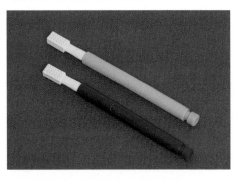

sensory system. Furthermore, this handy little rod also vibrates, which means that it can be used to create a powerful vibration stimulus as well as for the sensory perception of different surface structures. As a general rule, the tongue can and should be stimulated substantially and comprehensively. Stimulating the back third of the tongue is particularly effective in improving our interoceptive awareness, as this area is innervated by the vagus nerve.

The Z-Vibe has been specially designed to stimulate the oral cavity in order to improve interoceptive capacity.

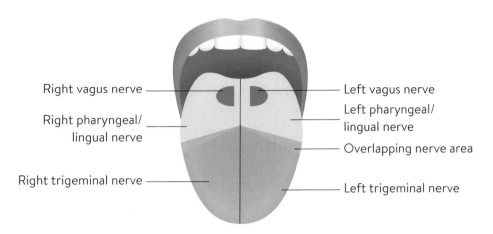

Right vagus nerve

Right pharyngeal/
lingual nerve

Right trigeminal nerve

Left vagus nerve

Left pharyngeal/
lingual nerve

Overlapping nerve area

Left trigeminal nerve

The tongue is supplied by various nerves. The back section, among other parts, is innervated by the vagus nerve.

1. Sit or stand in a comfortable position. Lengthen your spine but keep it nice and relaxed. Relax your head, neck and face, and allow your breath to flow smoothly and evenly. Open your mouth slightly and place the Z-Vibe on the right-hand side of your tongue, starting at the tip.

2. From here, slowly work your way to the back part. Then switch to the left-hand side of the tongue and repeat the stimulation from front to back. Focus on the way the vibration feels on your tongue. Where is it particularly noticeable? Where does it feel less intense? It's important that you keep checking and comparing which areas of the tongue you can feel more intensely and which ones you can't feel as well. The receptors that sense the vibration get tired very quickly. You should therefore switch to stimulating a new area every 10 to 15 seconds. Take care not to apply too much pressure and make sure the vibration of your tongue always feels comfortable.

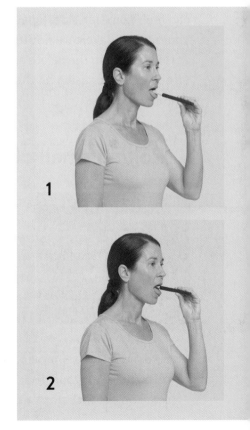

As we already mentioned, you can also focus on feeling the surface structure of the device. Noticing different structures not only increases your attention and concentration during the exercise, but also gives your brain another stimulus. This will make your training even more effective.

❯ Variation: Stimulating the oral cavity

The tongue is not the only part of the mouth that responds well to vibration. You can also use sensory stimulation on the roof of your mouth and your cheeks, which is particularly important as preparation for training the throat area.

Place the Z-Vibe in your mouth, slowly stroking it along your cheeks from back to front, starting with the right cheek and then the left. Compare how well you can feel it on each side. Finally, slowly stroke the Z-Vibe over the palate or roof of your mouth. Take care not to apply too much pressure and only move the Z-Vibe as far back along the palate as feels comfortable. To make your training even more effective, try focusing on the sensation of the surface structure too.

❯ Rolling small objects around in the mouth

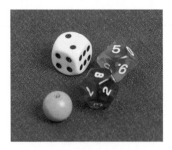

As an alternative to stimulating the tongue with the Z-Vibe, you can also try using dice, little balls or similar objects – as long as there is no risk of swallowing – for both sensory and motor stimulation of the tongue. The aim of this is to notice how the properties and structure of the various objects feel as you move them around your mouth and tongue.

1. Sit or stand in a comfortable position. Lengthen your spine but keep it nice and relaxed. Relax your neck, throat, jaw and face. Place a dice, marble or other small object with no sharp edges in your mouth.

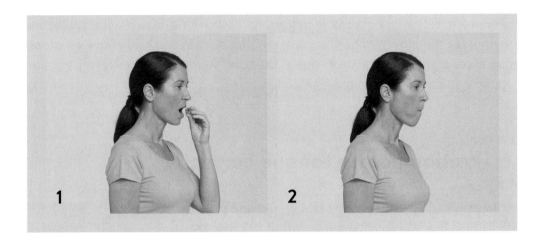

2. Slowly roll the object around your mouth for 2 to 3 minutes, noticing the way its shape, surface and structure feel on your tongue, palate and cheeks. Take your time! It is important to pay attention to how you perceive and feel the object. Can you feel it equally well on both sides of your tongue? Is it possible to move the object equally well around every area of your mouth? Change the items from time to time to keep your attention focused.

Tongue coordination

Improving the way your tongue moves is the main focus of the tongue training in this book. As we described at the start of this section, the tongue has a wide range of possible movements. The more successful you are at coordinating the tongue and accessing its full range of movement, the more information you will receive from this important organ, and the higher the quality of that information will be. Training the tongue is often extremely arduous when you first start, so make sure that you give yourself plenty of breaks and time to regenerate.

Build up your tongue training slowly and gently and don't overdo it. Start by optimising the basic positioning of your tongue. The sequence of the other tongue exercises is structured in such a way that you will require more and more coordination and control from one exercise to the next, as you gradually work towards achieving the right technique. Once you're confident that you've mastered the basic exercises, you may find it helpful to work with a metronome to set the rhythm for the movements. This gives you more focus and also activates important areas of the frontal lobe as well as the brain stem and midbrain, which makes your tongue training even more effective.

› **Positioning the tongue correctly**

The basic exercise for training the tongue is about learning how to assume and maintain the correct tongue position in the oral cavity. Having your tongue in the right position improves your breathing pattern, activates important cranial nerves and helps to increase the blood flow and activity levels in the insular cortex. It also helps to improve muscle tension in the neck and body, and therefore significantly increases the stability of the head and neck. Assuming the correct tongue position is also one of the simplest and most subtle training tools, which you can use several times a day to help you improve your interoceptive accuracy. Once you're confident that you can correctly adjust the basic position of your tongue, you should do so during respiratory training (pages 121–161) and when swallowing (pages 207–208) or gargling (pages 205–206). We strongly recommend that you also assume this tongue position during vestibular training (pages 66–85) and when mobilising the cervical spine (pages 98–101), as it makes these exercises more effective.

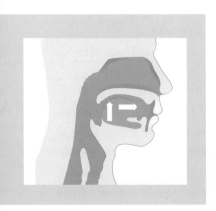

Sit or stand in a comfortable position. Lengthen your spine but keep it nice and relaxed. Relax your head, neck and jaw, and allow your breath to flow smoothly and evenly. Now focus your attention on the tip of your tongue and use it to touch your front incisors. From here, slide the tip of your tongue back towards your throat by about one centimetre, until you can feel a recess in the roof of your mouth. Place the tip of your tongue into this recess. From there, arch your entire tongue upwards onto the palate, applying a little pressure. Then push it gently and without any visible external movement towards the front of your mouth. Your tongue should not twist or shift, but should be in the same position on both sides. Take care to keep your face and jaw soft and relaxed, and gradually try to hold the tongue position with as little force and tension as possible.

❱ Tongue circles

Tongue circles is definitely the simplest and quickest way to create a lot of movement activity using your tongue. This activates and coordinates a large number of tongue muscles at once.

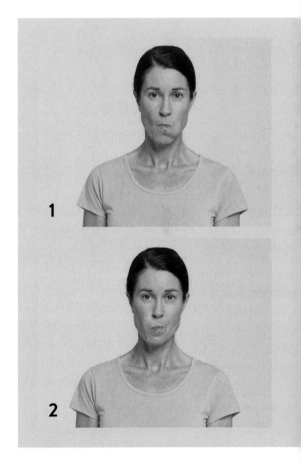

1. Stand or sit in a comfortable position. Lengthen your spine but keep it nice and relaxed. Relax your neck, face and jaw. Allow your breath to flow smoothly and evenly. Close your lips so that they are lightly touching and place the tip of your tongue in front of your incisors. Start to circle your tongue behind your closed lips.

2. Keep circling for six to ten rotations clockwise and another six to ten rotations anti-clockwise. Do the exercise slowly, really focusing your attention and keeping the movement controlled. Notice how the tongue, lips and teeth feel as your tongue makes the circling movements. Over time, try to make your circles bigger and bigger and to control the movement with the rear part of your tongue.

❱ Tongue side to side

Tongue movements from side to side can help to achieve a wider range of movement as you train your tongue. In contrast to tongue circles completing this
exercise properly requires more precision, control and concentration. Tongue
movements side to side not only add a new dimension to your training, but also
activate your insular cortex more extensively.

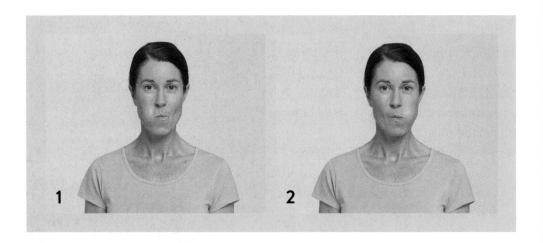

1. Sit or stand in a comfortable position. Lengthen your spine but keep it nice
   and relaxed. Relax your neck, face and jaw and hold your lips gently closed, but
   with your jaw slightly open. Allow your breath to flow smoothly and evenly.
   From this position, bring your tongue to your right cheek.
2. From here, move your tongue from cheek to cheek. Repeat this movement
   20 to 40 times. Make sure that your tongue stays horizontal throughout the
   exercise. Try to keep it parallel and avoid tilting or curling it. Imagine that your
   tongue is a tray that you mustn't tip over.

Note: Being aware of the position of your tongue is an important component
of this exercise. Once you've learned to keep your tongue parallel and relaxed,
feel free to vary the speed of the movement and the pressure you apply to your
cheeks.

❭ Pushing the tongue out and pulling it in

Similarly to moving your tongue sideways, pushing your tongue out and pulling in is another brilliant way to improve how well you can perceive and coordinate your tongue. Pushing your tongue out and pulling it in requires you to employ even more precision and control, as you have to keep the tongue parallel and symmetrical in order to do the movement correctly.

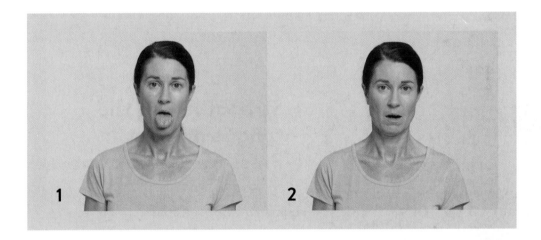

1. Sit or stand in a comfortable position. Lengthen your spine but keep it nice and relaxed. Relax your neck, spine, jaw and face, and allow your breath to flow smoothly and evenly. Open your mouth and jaw a little and start by pushing your tongue out as far as it will go.
2. Then pull your tongue as far back into your throat as it will go. Make sure that you keep your tongue parallel and wide as you push it out and in, keeping the movements even. Try not to curl it up or down or tilt it to either side. This requires a lot of control over the tongue muscles and undoubtedly takes a lot of practice at first. When you first start, you may wish to use a mirror to help you control the movement and the position of your tongue.

Strengthening the tongue

Alongside the coordination and control of its movement, another important element for improving the functionality of the tongue is to strengthen your tongue muscles. There are several factors that can cause some of your tongue muscles to be weaker than others, such as injuries, predominant use of one side of the tongue, slight misalignments in the jaw, as well as neurological factors such as the regulation of muscle tension or functional impairments in the cranial nerves that innervate the tongue. We will now show you a series of simple exercises that you can use to address these issues and strengthen the important muscles in your tongue.

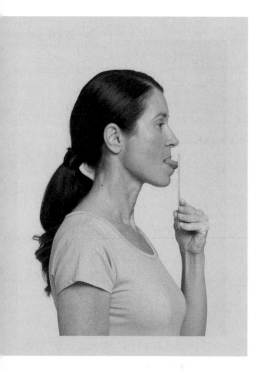

❯ Strengthening the tongue muscles 1: Pressure to the front

Equipment: Wooden stick

Sit or stand in a comfortable position. Lengthen your spine but keep it nice and relaxed. Relax your neck, throat, jaw and face, and allow your breath to flow smoothly and evenly. Stick your tongue out. Take a flat object such as a wooden stick or lollipop stick and press it gently against the end of your tongue from the front for 2 to 5 seconds. The key to this is not to apply so much pressure that the shape of your tongue changes. Relax your tongue fully and repeat the exercise five or six times in succession.

› Strengthening the tongue muscles 2: Pressure to the top and sides

Equipment: Wooden stick

1. Sit or stand in a comfortable position. Lengthen your spine but keep it nice and relaxed. Relax your neck, throat, jaw and face, and allow your breath to flow smoothly and evenly. From this position, stick your tongue out as far as you can. Take a flat object such as a wooden stick or lollipop stick and press it gently against the top of your tongue from above for 2 to 5 seconds. The key to this is not to apply so much pressure that your tongue moves or changes shape.
2. Then place the stick against the right side of your tongue and apply pressure against this part of the tongue for another 2 to 5 seconds.
3. Switch to the other side and place the object against the left side of your tongue, applying gentle pressure here for another 2 to 5 seconds. Relax your tongue fully and repeat the exercise five or six times.

Note: You can of course test and train each direction separately. Do more work with the directions in which you find yourself unable to create as much muscle tension.

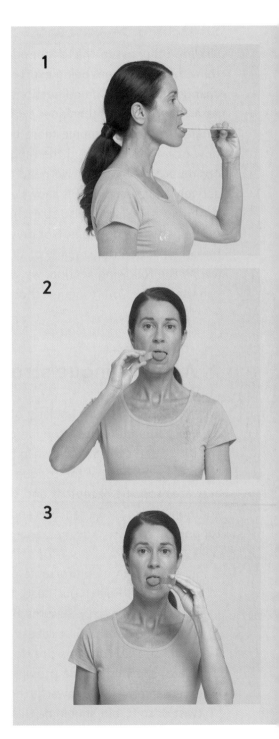

Stretching the tongue

Like any other tissue, the tongue adapts to whatever stresses it is regularly exposed to, with certain areas being exerted more and others less. This of course leads to changes and certain modifications in the tissues of the tongue. With active and passive stretching techniques, you can work specifically on those areas of the tongue that have become more tense and less mobile. In order to improve the flow of information from the range of different receptors in the tongue and to optimise their function, we need to be stretching our tongues regularly – both actively and passively. This allows us to activate specific receptors that only react to tensile stress, while also stretching the layers of fascial tissue and loosening up entire tissue connections. Not only does this make them work better, it also has a major impact on the stability of the neck and the position and movement of the jaw. In the following section, we will be showing you two simple techniques you can use to give your tongue a thorough, all-over stretch.

❯ Active tongue stretch

One exercise that's particularly effective is active stretching of the tongue. To do this, assume the basic tongue position described on pages 190–191. Opening the jaw initiates the stretch while the tongue stays in position. As well as actively stretching the base of the tongue and the connected fascial structures, this also activates specific receptors and strengthens specific muscles in the tongue. In addition, this exercise requires and improves your awareness and control of your tongue.

1. Sit or stand in a comfortable position. Lengthen your spine but keep it nice and relaxed. Relax your head, face and neck, and allow your breath to flow smoothly and evenly. Assume the natural tongue position by placing the tip of your tongue in the first recess in the roof of your mouth, keeping the shape symmetrical. From this position, arch your entire tongue upwards onto the palate, applying a little pressure. Then push it gently and without any visible external movement towards the front of your mouth. Your tongue should not twist or shift, but should be the same on both sides.

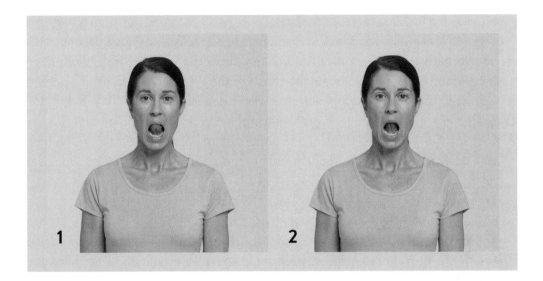

2. Open your mouth as wide as you can without changing the position of your tongue. Repeat this exercise eight to ten times, keeping the movement slow and controlled. Make sure that your tongue stays parallel to the roof of your mouth and try to open your jaw straight down without it shifting to either side.

› Passive tongue stretch

Equipment: Thin cloth

As well as actively stretching the tongue, it is also possible to stretch it passively. Passive stretching offers a wider variety of ways to stretch the different sections and structures of your tongue. We will now show you an easy way to stretch the most important areas of your tongue. All you need is a cloth to allow you to hold and move your tongue in a safe and controlled manner. The tongue is very delicate and sensitive, so do these stretches slowly and carefully. Give yourself plenty of time to get a feel for the tension in this sensitive area.

1. Sit or stand in a comfortable position. Lengthen your spine but keep it nice and relaxed. Make sure your neck, jaw and face are as relaxed as possible, and allow your breath to flow smoothly and evenly. Take the cloth in your hand, open your mouth and hold your tongue through the cloth, applying even pressure with your thumb, index finger and middle finger.

2. From here, carefully pull your whole tongue forwards and slightly upwards so that you feel a gentle stretch on the underside of your tongue. Start by holding this stretch for 30 to 60 seconds, and gradually build that up to 2 to 5 minutes over time.

3. Then pull your tongue slightly towards the right from the centre.

4. Then pull it slightly towards the left from the centre.

5. Then stretch the tongue upwards slightly. If there are directions in which you feel more tension from the stretch, hold these stretches for a little longer. Stretch your tongue in these positions for between 30 seconds and 5 minutes in total. You may wish to repeat the whole exercise two or three times.

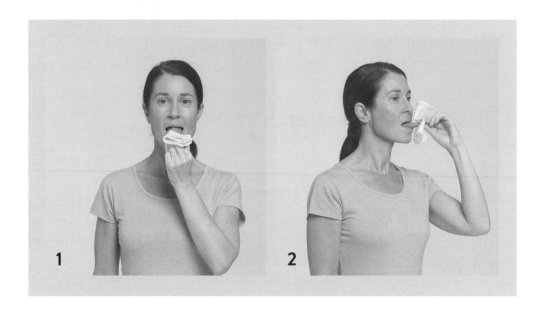

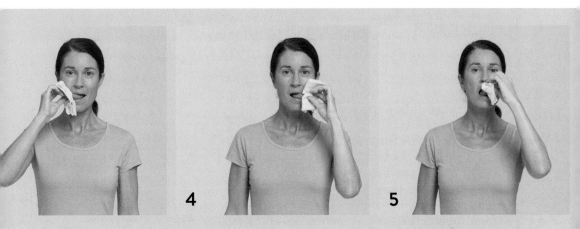

Categorising the tongue training exercises			
Exercise	Positive	Neutral/moderately positive	Save for later
Improving awareness of the tongue with stimulation (pages 186–189)			
Sensory stimulation of the tongue using the Z-Vibe (pages 186–187)			
Variation: Stimulating the oral cavity (page 188)			
Rolling small objects around in the mouth (pages 188–189)			
Tongue coordination (pages 189–193)			
Positioning the tongue correctly (pages 190–191)			
Tongue circles (page 191)			

Categorising the tongue training exercises			
Exercise	Positive	Neutral/moderately positive	Save for later
Tongue coordination (pages 189–193)			
Tongue side to side (page 192)			
Pushing the tongue out and pulling it in (page 193)			
Strengthening the tongue (pages 194–195)			
Strengthening the tongue muscles 1: Pressure to the front (page 194)			
Strengthening the tongue muscles 2: Pressure to the top and sides (page 195)			
Stretching the tongue (pages 196–199)			
Active tongue stretch (pages 196–197)			
Passive tongue stretch (pages 197–199)			

Recommendations for tongue training

The tongue exercises can be carried out in a range of different ways. The first option would be to use them to do standalone tongue training sessions in order to hone your interoceptive awareness over several weeks. Tongue exercises are particularly effective at activating the posterior section of your insular cortex and therefore help to alleviate digestion and pelvic floor problems. Intensive tongue training also improves core stability and has positive effects on breathing, vocal training and the stability of your head and neck. So, if you've found the tongue exercises work well for you or, alternatively, you have found them very difficult, you should focus on this aspect of the interoceptive awareness training for about three to six weeks. This will help you to achieve a powerful and lasting activation of the insular cortex, and you will benefit from all the other positive effects mentioned too.

The second option would be to use the tongue training as part of your wider interoceptive awareness training. In this case, you would incorporate the tongue exercises into your daily routine, doing them several times a day in order to experience their many positive effects. This is the perfect approach if you're simply looking to improve your overall wellbeing and interoceptive awareness.

The third option would be to use tongue exercises as a warm-up for other aspects of your interoceptive awareness training. Practical application of this powerful and unique form of stimulation shows that it often significantly increases the effectiveness and sustainability of the training.

Tongue exercises as the main element of your training

You will probably find that exercising the tongue muscles is more challenging and requires more focus and attention than you may have initially imagined. We therefore recommend that you limit your training to just a few minutes a day to begin with. Start with 3 to 5 minutes, three or four times a day, and gradually build up to a total of 20 to 30 minutes of training a day.

In practice, evidence shows that starting your tongue training with sensory exercises, i.e. those that focus on touch and feel, is extremely effective. To warm up for your training, start by stimulating your tongue with the Z-Vibe (pages 186–187) or by rolling a small object around in your mouth (pages 188–189). You will find that this enables you to perform any subsequent tongue exercises much more efficiently and precisely. After that, work on coordinating and strengthening the tongue muscles. Tongue circles (page 191) makes a great starting point as it acutely activates all the relevant muscles. Then choose two or three more tongue exercises from the categories 'tongue coordination' (pages 189–193) and 'strengthening the tongue' (pages 194–195) for which you had a positive or neutral assessment result. Do these for a few minutes. Finally, if necessary, do some active or passive tongue stretch (pages 196–199).

You can and should switch up the exercises as you wish, in order to make the training more varied. For the best possible results, keep practising the tongue training for several weeks.

Tongue exercises as part of interoceptive awareness training

Although we do advise that you'll get the best results from doing a sensory warm-up before the tongue exercises, it's also fine to simply incorporate your tongue training into everyday life without doing a warm-up. Choose a variety of tongue coordination, strengthening and stretching exercises for which you had a positive assessment result, and do them two to three times a day for 1 to 2 minutes.

Tongue exercises as a warm-up for other training

Because the tongue has such a powerful and unique capacity to stimulate the brain and nervous system, tongue training is also ideal as a warm-up for vestibular training, respiratory training and pelvic floor training. To do this, choose two to three tongue exercises for which you had a positive assessment result and do these for 30 seconds to 1 minute before starting your other training. Of course, a short 10 to 20-second sensory stimulation will also make these tongue exercises more effective.

Recommendations for tongue training		
Potential use	Scope and application	Effect
As the main element of the training	**Sensory warm-up** Spend 1 or 2 minutes on one of the following exercises: • Sensory stimulation with the Z-Vibe (pages 186–187) • Rolling small objects around in the mouth (pages 188–189) **Global activation** Tongue circles (page 191), 5 to 15 rotations in each direction	• Intensely stimulates the posterior section of the insular cortex • The exercises for tongue coordination and strengthening the tongue also activate the anterior section of the insular cortex • Improves: • digestive problems

Recommendations for tongue training		
Potential use	**Scope and application**	**Effect**

As the main element of the training	**Main section**
	• 2 to 3 tongue coordination and strengthening exercises with positive assessment results
	• Carry out for 2 to 4 minutes, using a metronome if you wish
	• Finish off with a tongue stretching exercise if required
	
	• Start with 3 to 5 minutes on each, 3 or 4 times per day
	• Increase this to 15 to 20 minutes per day, in 2 or 3 sessions
	• Carry out over the course of 3 to 4 weeks
		• Improves:
		  • pelvic floor problems
		  • interoceptive awareness
		  • general wellbeing and fitness
		  • core stability and posture by activating the supplementary motor areas

As part of interoceptive awareness training	• 1 to 3 exercises with positive assessment results • 1 to 2 minutes • 2 to 3 times per day	
As a warm-up for other training exercises	• 2 to 3 exercises with positive assessment results • Do these for 30 to 60 seconds each	Particularly suitable as a warm-up for: • vestibular training • respiratory training • pelvic floor training

Throat exercises to stimulate the pharyngeal branches of the vagus nerve

The area of the throat innervated by the vagus nerve is not restricted to the tongue. There are also branches of the vagus nerve in the back of the oral cavity and the throat. Like the tongue, the throat area is extensively represented in the brain, with a large area allocated to it. The oral cavity and throat, like the tongue, constitute an internal structure. Training this area is therefore fundamental to improving your interoceptive awareness.

The signals that run through the throat area to the insular cortex are predominantly processed in the posterior section, so these exercises work particularly well for alleviating physical problems, especially those related to your digestion. The back of the oral cavity and the lower throat can be controlled through a series of simple, everyday exercises such as gargling, humming, swallowing and sensory stimulation using different water temperatures.

❭ Humming

Humming acutely activates the area right at the back of the oral cavity and deep down in the throat, as well as the vagus nerve. There are various ways in which we can use humming to help improve our interoceptive awareness, and they can be done anywhere. Humming for at least 10 minutes activates the parasympathetic nervous system and helps to reduce feelings of anxiety. Plus, it can be a lot of fun! For example, you can hum along to the radio as you drive to work in the morning, or hum while you're in the shower or similar situations to activate your insular cortex. Use the time you already have as effectively as possible, and be creative! As a general rule, humming should be done with the tongue in the natural position as described on pages 190–191.

Sit or stand in a comfortable position. Lengthen your spine but keep it nice and relaxed. Allow your breath to flow smoothly and evenly. Roll in your head slightly, lowering your nose by 1 or 2 cm keeping your neck nice and relaxed. If you've already got the hang of it, assume the correct tongue position (pages 190–191). From this position, start by humming for around 10 to 30 seconds. It's not a problem if, at first, you find you occasionally have to stop humming and then start again. This is completely normal and will improve over time.

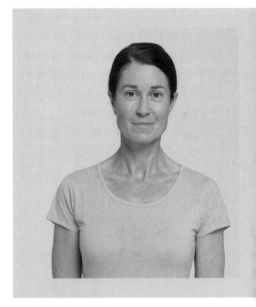

Then focus your attention on the back of your throat and how the vibration created by your humming feels there. Does the humming feel the same on both sides? Does it seem louder on one side than on the other? If the humming feels more noticeable on one side, then we would recommend that you focus more on the side where the humming is less noticeable. To do this, simply focus your attention specifically on this side.

❯ Variation: Humming at different pitches

It's really easy to create infinite variations of this exercise. All you have to do is change your pitch while you're humming. Do the exercise as described earlier, but this time mix things up by humming at a lower or higher pitch. Varying your voice and pitch is one of the simplest and most effective throat exercises there is. As well as being easy and fun, it targets the branches of the vagus nerve located there.

❯ Gargling

Equipment: A glass of still water

As with humming, gargling has a powerful stimulatory effect on your interoceptive system. Firstly, the vagus nerve itself is involved in the process of gargling, and secondly, simply noticing the movement of the structures involved, as well as the feel of the water, its movement, consistency and temperature is in itself an interoceptive process. As simple as this exercise may initially sound, many people find gargling surprisingly difficult. If, contrary to expectations, you find it difficult to gargle water, we recommend that you start by warming up the back of your mouth and the muscles required for gargling for 20 to 30 seconds beforehand. The following exercises work well: Tongue circles (page 191), stimulating the tongue using the Z-Vibe (pages 186–187), humming (pages 204–205) and vibrating the front teeth (page 110).

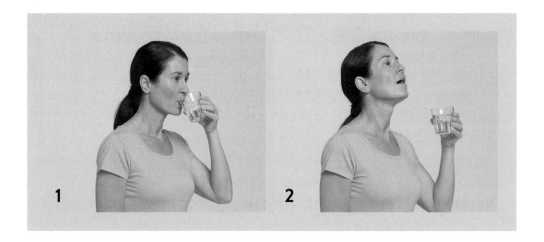

1. Stand or sit in a comfortable position. Lengthen your spine but keep it nice and relaxed. Allow your breath to flow evenly. Take a small sip of water and hold it in your mouth.
2. Now tilt your head back and start gargling. Continue gargling for 10 to 20 seconds. It's absolutely fine if occasionally you need to take a break and then start again. When doing this exercise, make sure that you only tilt your head as far back as is comfortable. Once you have practised a little more, shift your attention towards how the gargling feels. Notice whether it feels the same on both sides, or if one side seems to be doing more of the work. If you notice that one side is doing more of the work, gradually try to bring the movement over to the other side of the throat.

❯ Variation: Gargling with different water temperatures

Equipment: Several glasses of still water at different temperatures

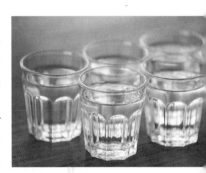

With this variation, you gargle with water at various different temperatures, one after the other. Noticing the different temperatures increases the range of sensations and therefore activates the sensory components of your interoceptive system more intensely. Gargling with different water temperatures not only trains your movement and coordination, but also your perception of temperature, which also activates the insular cortex. Make sure that the water temperatures stay within a range that you're comfortable with.

Part-fill one glass with warm water and another with cold. Stand or sit in a comfortable position. Lengthen your spine but keep it nice and relaxed. Take a small sip from the first glass and hold the water in your mouth. Now tilt your head back and start gargling. Continue gargling for 10 to 20 seconds, then spit out the water and move on to the next glass. Focus on feeling the movement and temperature of the water in your throat. Pay attention to whether you are able to sense the different water temperatures equally well on both sides of your throat. Do the coldness and warmth of the water feel the same on both the right and left sides of your throat? Is it more difficult to feel the water temperature on one side? If you do notice differences here, we recommend focusing more of your attention on the side that is less sensitive.

❯ Swallowing

Equipment: A glass of still water

As with humming and gargling, swallowing is also an extremely intensive interoceptive process. Like gargling, many people find it really quite difficult. In normal circumstances, you should be able to take four or five 'dry' swallows in quick succession at any time. In other words, you would be able to swallow without drinking any liquid. Is this the case for you? When you first start working on the swallowing motion, we recommend you begin by swallowing liquid as it makes the process much easier. If you do find swallowing difficult, it helps to warm up for this exercise by circling the tongue (page 191), stimulating the tongue using the Z-Vibe (pages 186–187), humming (pages 204–205) and vibrating the front teeth (page 110). A brief run-through of the recommended exercises – say around 20 to 30 seconds – is plenty. As a general rule, you can and should do the swallowing exercise with your tongue in the natural position (pages 190–191).

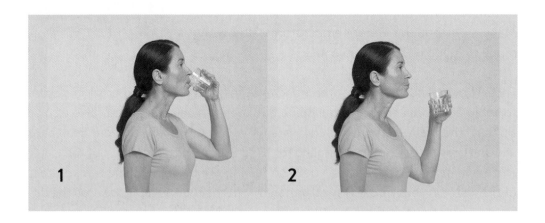

1. Sit or stand in a comfortable position. Lengthen your spine but keep it nice and relaxed. Allow your breath to flow smoothly and evenly. Take a small sip of water and hold it in your mouth. If you've already got the hang of it, assume the correct tongue position.
2. Try to use as many individual swallowing motions as possible to swallow that one sip of water. Repeat this process several times in succession, until you have done a total of 10 to 20 swallows. Once you have got the hang of it, try to notice how the water feels and whether one side of your throat seems to play a larger or smaller role in the swallowing process. If you notice that one side seems weaker, focus more on integrating that side into the swallowing process.

Categorising the exercises that activate the throat area			
Exercise	Positive	Neutral/moderately positive	Save for later
Humming (pages 204–205)			
Variation: Humming at different pitches (page 205)			
Gargling (pages 205–206)			
Variation: Gargling with different water temperatures (page 207)			
Swallowing (pages 207–208)			

Training recommendations for activating the vagus nerve in the mouth and throat

As with tongue training, there are three ways in which you can approach training the interoceptive components located in the mouth and throat: as the main focus of your training, as one part of a more comprehensive training plan, or as a warm-up for exercises focusing on other areas. The approach you choose depends on what you want to achieve. Stimulating the branches of the vagus nerve in the throat area specifically activates the posterior section of the insular cortex. Using the mouth and throat exercises for standalone training sessions is therefore particularly useful if you want to address symptoms that are more physical in nature, such as problems with digestion. If you make humming (pages 204–205) the focus of your training, this taps into your parasympathetic nervous system and helps to reduce the symptoms of anxiety and depressive moods.

You can also use the exercises that activate the branches of the vagus nerve in your throat as a partial element of your interoceptive awareness training. With this approach, the exercises should be spread out in short sessions throughout the course of the day. You should combine these exercises with exercises focusing on other elements of your interoceptive awareness, to make a total daily training duration of 20 to 30 minutes. Of course, you can also use the effects of the throat exercises as a warm-up for other exercises.

Throat exercises as the main element of your training

As with tongue training, evidence shows that a quick sensory warm-up increases the effectiveness of exercises designed to activate the vagus nerve in the throat area. Start by stimulating the mouth and throat area with the Z-Vibe or a similar device (page 188), or choose one or two tongue exercises (pages 191–199) that work particularly well for you. It is also very helpful to vibrate the incisors for 10 to 20 seconds (page 110). You will then find it much easier to coordinate your throat in any subsequent exercises. Make sure that you move on to the exercises focusing on specific structures of the throat as soon as you finish your warm-up. Choose exercises for which you had a positive or neutral assessment result and repeat this training two to three times a day. You can and should switch up the exercises as you wish, in order to vary your training and make it different each time. Like the tongue training, you should persevere with the exercises focusing on the structures in the throat area for three to four weeks to achieve the best and most lasting effects.

Throat exercises as part of interoceptive awareness training

The throat exercises can also fit easily into your daily routine without you having to do any sensory warm-ups. To do this, carry out one of the specified exercises two or three times a day for 1 to 2 minutes. Try gargling with lukewarm water after you've brushed your teeth, humming in the shower or singing along to the radio in the car. You could also get into the habit of really paying attention as you take the first few sips of a drink, and making sure your tongue is in the right position.

Throat exercises as a warm-up for other training exercises

Activating the throat area also makes a great warm-up for tongue exercises and pelvic floor training. Choose two or three of the throat activation exercises and spend 30 to 60 seconds on them before your main training.

Training recommendations for activating the vagus nerve in the mouth and throat		
Potential use	**Scope and application**	**Effect**

As the main element of the training	**Sensory warm-up**
	Spend 1 or 2 minutes on one of the following exercises:
	• Sensory stimulation of the tongue using the Z-Vibe (pages 186–187), plus the variation involving stimulation of the oral cavity (page 188)
	• Vibrating the front teeth (page 110)
	• 1 tongue exercise with positive assessment result
	
	Main section
	• 2 to 3 exercises with positive assessment results
	• 3 to 5 minutes (starting with 2 to 3 minutes)
	• 2 to 3 times throughout the day
	• Carry out over the course of 3 to 4 weeks
		• Activates the posterior section of the insular cortex
		• Improves:
		   • digestive disorders
		   • anxiety and depressive moods, for which prolonged humming works particularly well (pages 204–205)

As part of general interoceptive awareness training	• 1 to 2 exercises with positive assessment results • 1 to 2 minutes • 2 to 3 times per day	
As a warm-up for other training exercises	• 2 to 3 exercises with positive assessment results • Do these for 30 to 60 seconds each	Particularly suitable as a warm-up for: • tongue exercises • pelvic floor training

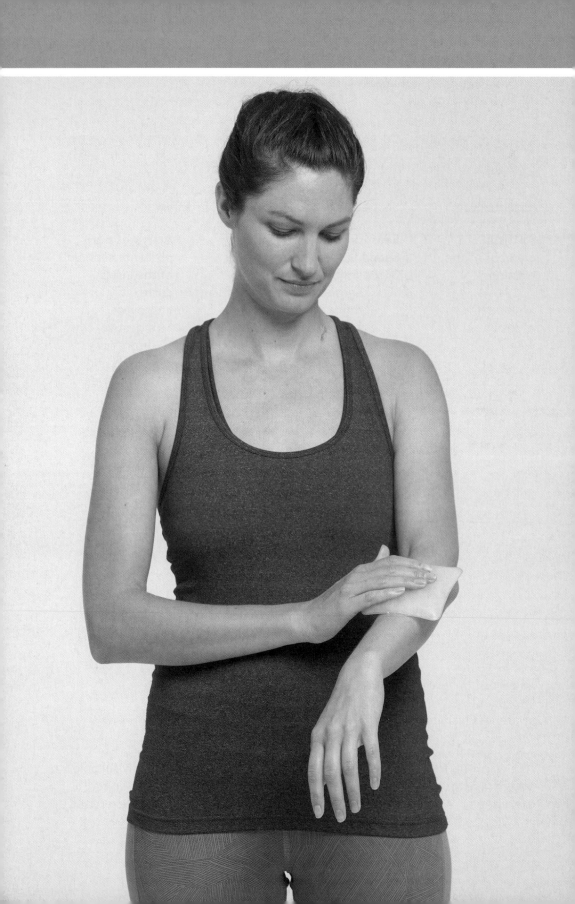

6

Touch, sound and vision for better interoceptive awareness

The importance of all five senses

We often only become aware of how important our sensory perceptions are for our daily lives, our fitness and our health when one of them no longer works properly. Our modern lifestyle plays a major role in the deterioration of our senses. This in turn reduces our general capacity for information processing, including our ability to process information from within our own bodies. As you saw in Chapter 1 on pages 10 to 29, our brains need all the information from our surroundings, our movements and our interoceptive awareness in order to adjust the autonomic nervous system according to our perception of the overall situation. This information determines how the sympathetic and parasympathetic nervous systems should respond to the situation. You may remember that the regulation of the relationship between the 'fight or flight' nerves and the 'rest and digest' nerves within the autonomic nervous system is an output of the insular cortex.

To round off the range of topics, this chapter is dedicated to improving the specific aspects of touch and hearing that influence our interoceptive awareness. We will also be looking at how to activate the parasympathetic nervous system by relaxing our eyes. The elements covered here, such as localising and differentiating acoustic signals and noticing differences in pressure and temperature, are things that often get neglected amongst the hubbub of daily life. Improving the quality of the information received from our senses of touch, hearing and sight, which is essential for our interoceptive awareness, activates the insular cortex and helps to improve our interoceptive accuracy. The comprehensive integration of these senses is another key factor in achieving the greatest degree of interoceptive awareness, and is therefore the foundation of health and fitness.

In the following section, we will be covering those areas of our perception in which information is transmitted that directly affects the activity level of the insular cortex, and therefore impacts our interoceptive awareness. Firstly, we will look at the concept of 'C fibres', which are activated when we perceive different temperatures and pressure applied to our skin and internal organs. C fibres are special nerve fibres that can transmit different types of information due to their free nerve endings. Similar to the vagus nerve, they deliver a vast quantity of sensory information to the posterior section of the insular cortex and therefore have the capacity for acute and targeted activation of this area.

We will then look more closely at one particular aspect of our hearing – that of localising and differentiating acoustic signals in the space around us. This activates specific areas within the central section of the insular cortex, in which this information is processed. This improves the process of integration within the insular cortex and therefore optimises the overall effect of the training, as well as your interoceptive awareness. As we come to the end of the chapter, we will show you a series of simple eye relaxation exercises to activate your parasympathetic nervous system. This is a quick and easy way to reduce your stress levels.

Perceiving temperature differences

It is extremely important for our bodies to be able to regulate temperature. Without the ability to control body temperature properly – a process that happens completely autonomously – we simply wouldn't survive. It is essential for maintaining the entire metabolism of an organism. As already described in Chapter 1 on pages 23 and 25, the part of the brain responsible for this is the thermosensory cortex, located in the posterior section of the insular cortex. It receives and evaluates information about our temperature from the thermal receptors located in the skin. Considering the functions of the insular cortex, it makes perfect sense that it is involved in the perception and regulation of body temperature.

You can consciously activate the thermosensory cortex by applying moderate heat or cold to parts of your body. You can use hot and cold packs for this, or simply rub your hands together until they are warm and then place them on one area of your skin. Touching metal objects or showering at different temperatures also activates these specific thermoreceptors. Applying heat and cold over an extended period of time is an easy and effective way to create high levels of activity in the insular cortex. Wearing an abdominal belt (page 222) has been found to be an ideal way of attaching hot or cold packs to the body. Exercises based on the perception of different temperatures can be combined with other activities designed to improve interoceptive awareness, such as breathing or pelvic floor exercises, to increase the overall effectiveness of the training.

❯ Sensing heat and cold

Equipment: A hot water bottle, warm wheat bag or heat pack, plus a cold pack

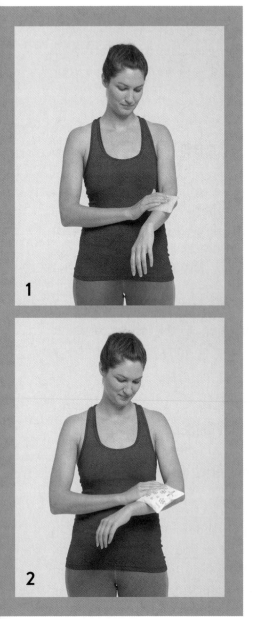

A simple and effective way to expose the body to different temperatures and activate the thermoregulatory responses is to apply or rub hot or cold objects onto the body. Use any items you have available to you to apply the different temperatures, then focus on how they feel. For example, hot water bottles, microwavable pillows, cold packs or cool drinks bottles all work well.

1. Sit, stand or lie in a comfortable position. Lengthen your spine but keep it nice and relaxed. Allow your breath to flow smoothly and evenly. Choose a heat pack, such as a hot water bottle or warm wheat bag. Stroke this gently over your left arm for 30 to 60 seconds, applying just a little pressure, then over your left leg. Try to consciously notice how the warmth feels. Then switch sides and stroke it slowly and gently along your right arm and leg for 30 to 60 seconds each. Does the heat feel the same on your left and right sides? Does the sensation of the heat feel more or less intense on different areas of one arm or leg? Switch to the torso and apply the heat pack in turn to your stomach, chest and back. How does the heat feel in these areas?

2. Then switch to the cold pack and use the same method to apply it to the different parts of your body. The cold pack should be cool, rather than being uncomfortably cold.

❯ Variation: Applying the heat and cold for longer

Another way to tap into your body's perception of different temperatures is to leave the warm or cold objects on an area of your body for longer. You should only do this if it works well for you and if applying heat and cold gives you a positive assessment result. Activating the posterior section of the insular cortex this intensely and for this long improves your general interoceptive awareness and helps to regulate stress. Applying heat to the abdomen, in particular, supports the parasympathetic nervous system and aids relaxation.

Categorising the application of heat and cold			
Exercise	Positive	Neutral/moderately positive	Save for later
Sensing heat and cold (page 216)			
Sensing heat			
Sensing cold			
Variation: Applying the heat and cold for longer (see above)			
Applying the heat for longer			
Applying the cold for longer			

Training recommendations for perceiving heat and cold

As with the other exercises in this book, you can easily build the heat and cold perception exercises into your daily routine. This way, you can train your interoceptive awareness and exercise your insular cortex with almost no effort whatsoever. If you want to work on improving this aspect of your interoceptive awareness exclusively, you should aim to do 10 to 15 minutes of training per day. Heat and cold treatment is particularly effective for acute activation of the posterior section of the insular cortex, and has a positive effect on pain patterns and emotional regulation. The use of heat in particular often provides even better results.

If you find that the application and perception of different temperatures works really well for you, you can try applying the hot and cold packs for even longer – between 20 and 30 minutes. Simply tie a heat pad or cooling pad to your stomach while doing normal everyday activities such as household chores, working at the computer, watching TV or reading. You could also try putting a hot water bottle on your stomach before going to sleep at night.

The perception of different temperatures can also be used as a quick way to activate the insular cortex between other activities, in order to pad out your general interoceptive awareness training. The ultimate goal is to improve your general health and interoceptive accuracy. To do this, simply build 1 or 2 minutes of temperature perception into your daily routine, two to three times a day. As always, it is important that you spend a total of at least 20 minutes a day training your insular cortex. The perception of temperature differences also works well as a warm-up for other exercises. To do this, simply spend 1 to 2 minutes applying and perceiving heat and cold, thus activating the posterior section of the insular cortex and making any subsequent exercises more effective.

Combine the exercises with one another

Experiment with combining exercises based on perceiving different temperatures with other exercises that stimulate the insular cortex. This reinforces the positive impact of the individual exercises. If you combine several exercises at once, not only does this intensify the level of stimulation in the brain, but adapting to different stimuli also increases the overall effect of the training. More information can be found in Chapter 8 from page 263 onwards. Here are a few examples of possible combinations for heat application:

- Wear a heat pad underneath your abdominal belt (page 222).

- Perform a deep pressure massage using warm massage oil to increase your interoceptive awareness (pages 220–221).

• Combine heat application with the breathing exercises on page 123 onwards, as well as the pelvic floor exercises on pages 170 to 177 in Chapter 4. Place a hot water bottle or heat pad on your stomach while you carry out breathing or pelvic floor exercises.

When combining the application of heat or cold with other exercises, we recommend regularly turning your focus to how the temperature feels throughout the exercise. For example, you might shift your attention away from your breathing or your pelvic floor muscles for a moment to notice how the heat or cold feels. Shifting your attention in this way forces your brain to integrate the sensation of the heat more rigorously, thus increasing the benefits of the exercise.

Training recommendations for perceiving heat and cold		
Potential use	**Scope and application**	**Effect**

As the main element of the training	• 10 to 15 minutes of hot and cold sensory exercises
	• 20 to 30 minutes per day, if you notice a benefit
		• Activates the posterior section of the insular cortex
		• Improves:
		  • chronic pain
		  • depressive moods
		  • anxiety

As part of interoceptive awareness training	• 1 to 2 minutes • 2 to 3 times per day	
As a warm-up for other training exercises	• 1 to 2 minutes of hot or cold sensory exercises • Pick the variation for which you got the best assessment results	• Activates the posterior section of the insular cortex • Improves the overall effectiveness of the training
In combination with other exercises	Options • Secure heat pads beneath the abdominal belt	• Activates the posterior section of the insular cortex

Training recommendations for perceiving heat and cold		
Potential use	Scope and application	Effect

	• Use warm oil for pressure massage
	• Apply hot water bottle or heat pads to the stomach while doing breathing or pelvic floor exercises
		• Improves:
		  • chronic pain
		  • digestive disorders
		  • emotional regulation
		  • anxiety
		  • depressive moods
		  • pelvic floor problems

Pressure and deep tissue massage

Other important areas that are innervated by the vagus nerve and the C fibres, with their free nerve endings, are the rib cage and the internal organs (see the figure on page 18 that illustrates the route of the vagus nerve). This makes pressure massage and other forms of applying pressure to the chest and abdominal area particularly effective. Massaging these areas activates the vagus nerve as well as a number of C fibres, sending a vast quantity of sensory information to the posterior section of the insular cortex.

Light pressure massage

The following exercises involve massaging the chest and stomach with a little more pressure for 3 to 5 minutes. You may wish to use a warm massage oil for an even greater effect on the insular cortex. If you find this pressure massage works well for you, feel free to repeat it two or three times a day.

❯ Massaging the chest

Lie or sit in a comfortable position. Lengthen your spine but keep it nice and relaxed. Allow your breath to flow smoothly and evenly. Using either your thumbs or your index and middle fingers, start by massaging your chest muscles for 2 to 3 minutes. Use small, circular strokes or run your fingers horizontally from your breast bone in the middle of your rib cage towards your armpits. Make sure that you massage every little section of your chest muscles. Start with light to medium pressure. If it feels good, try increasing the pressure. However, it should always stay within a range that feels comfortable.

Note: Using the assessments, test which intensity works best for you and your nervous system. The mobility assessments (Chapter 2, pages 36–39) and pain level assessments (Chapter 2, pages 40–41) work particularly well.

❯ Massaging the abdominal area

Lie or sit in a comfortable resting position. Lengthen your spine but keep it nice and relaxed. Allow your breath to flow smoothly and evenly. Massage your stomach for 3 to 5 minutes. Try placing your index, middle and ring fingers together on each hand and then laying them on top of one another. This will distribute the pressure more evenly and allow you to use the force of both hands. As with the chest massage, it helps to use small, circular movements. Make sure that you cover the whole of your abdominal area. Start with light to medium pressure and gradually increase it. The pressure should always be within a range that's comfortable for you.

Note: Using the assessments, test which intensity works best for you and your nervous system. The mobility assessments (Chapter 2, pages 36–39) and pain level assessments (Chapter 2, pages 40–41) work really well for this.

❯ Wearing an abdominal belt

Equipment: Abdominal belt

As well as massage, you can also use an elasticated abdominal belt to apply pressure to the stomach area. The tension in the belt stimulates the skin and muscles and applies pressure to the internal organs, both of which activate the C fibres, with their free nerve endings. The pressure also activates the vagus nerve. Wearing an abdominal belt is therefore a very effective way of sending a large quantity of interoceptive information to the insular cortex. It also enables prolonged stimulation of the C fibres. This simple, straightforward and inconspicuous method therefore allows you to initiate prolonged activation of the insular cortex with no additional effort. Abdominal belts are very versatile and efficient – you can wear one in your spare time, while at work or to further increase the effectiveness of your training.

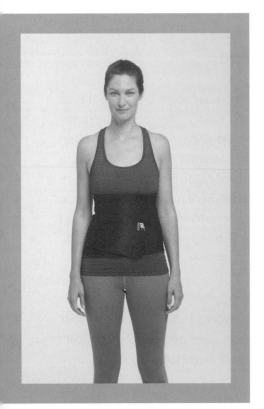

Stand with your feet hip-width apart. Lengthen your spine but keep it nice and relaxed. Allow your breath to flow smoothly and evenly. Pull the abdominal belt tightly around your stomach. Make sure that the belt is pulled taut, but not so tight that it feels uncomfortable to wear. You can wrap the abdominal belt round your stomach in either direction. We often find that one direction gets better results than the other. Use the assessments to work out which direction works best for you. You can wear the belt for between 20 minutes and 2 hours at a time. Feel free to put it on two or three times a day.

Categorising the application of pressure and deep massage			
Exercise	Positive	Neutral/ moderately positive	Save for later
Light pressure massage (pages 220–222)			
Massaging the chest (page 221)			
Massaging the abdominal area (page 221)			
Wearing an abdominal belt (page 222)			
Wrapped clockwise around the abdomen			
Wrapped anti-clockwise around the abdomen			

Training recommendations for the application of pressure and deep massage

To activate the C fibres through deep pressure massage, we recommend you dedicate at least 5 to 10 minutes a day to the massage. To really feel the effects of wearing the abdominal belt, you should wear it for at least 20 minutes a day. Practice has shown that the best and most lasting results are achieved by wearing the abdominal belt for several hours at a time. Because it's so simple to use, the abdominal belt is ideal for combining with other elements of your training. Try wearing it while you're doing your tongue, breathing, pelvic floor or vestibular exercises to optimise the effects of your training on the insular cortex.

Training recommendations for the application of pressure and deep massage		
Potential use	Scope and application	Effect

As the main element of the training	• 1 exercise with positive assessment result from:
	  • massaging the chest (page 221)
	  • massaging the abdominal area (page 221)
	• At least 10 minutes of massage per day
		• Activates the posterior section of the insular cortex
		• Improves:
		  • digestive problems
		  • emotional regulation
		  • anxiety
		  • depressive moods

For continued activation	Wear the abdominal belt for between 20 minutes and several hours	
As part of interoceptive awareness training, in combination with other exercises	Wear the abdominal belt during: • respiratory training • tongue exercises • pelvic floor training • vestibular training	• Activates the posterior section of the insular cortex • Enhances the effect of the training

Acoustic mapping

Our ability to perceive and accurately identify sounds from our surroundings is crucial to our safety and survival. If the brain is unable to perceive and assess where noises and sounds come from and what they mean, then it has a shortage of the extremely important information that is required for interoception and sensory integration. Localising sounds and pitches activates the central section of the insular cortex, as this is where any elements of acoustic signal processing are evaluated and integrated.

This part of the brain is also involved in our ability to localise, perceive and process sounds of different frequencies (pitches). Localising the source of a sound is crucial to our orientation and enables us to make a safe assessment of our surroundings. It also has a positive effect on memory and even improves the stability of the spine and body. Poor orientation goes hand in hand with poor interoceptive awareness. The following exercises will allow you to activate this specific area in the central section of the insular cortex, which will increase your ability to interpret and integrate information from inside your body. The improvement in acoustic orientation will also help to stabilise your body and reduce your stress levels.

❯ Localising sounds

Localising acoustic signals is a simple and fun way to tap into the central section of the insular cortex and improve the integration of sensory data. All you need is a training partner to make the sounds for you and give you feedback on your accuracy.

1. Stand or sit in a comfortable position. Lengthen your spine but keep it nice and relaxed. Allow your breath to flow smoothly and evenly. Have your training partner stand about 1.5 to 2 m away from you. Close your eyes, relax and tune your hearing into the space around you. Your training partner will now click their fingers.
2. Point to the exact point where you think the noise came from, i.e. where the hand clicked.
3. Keep your finger pointed towards the source of the sound and open your eyes to check if you were right.
4. If you were wrong, move your hand so that you're pointing directly at the correct location. Then close your eyes again and your partner will click in a different place. Carry out this exercise for 3 to 5 minutes. It's important that your training partner uses all areas of the space over the course of the exercise – top right and left, bottom right and left, and top and bottom in the middle. Is there an area where you find it harder to localise the sound? If so, try to focus more on this area in your training.

❯ Variation: Varying the volume

To mix your training up a bit and make it more efficient, you can try varying the volume of the clicking. This often makes localising the sound much more difficult and improves your focus and concentration.

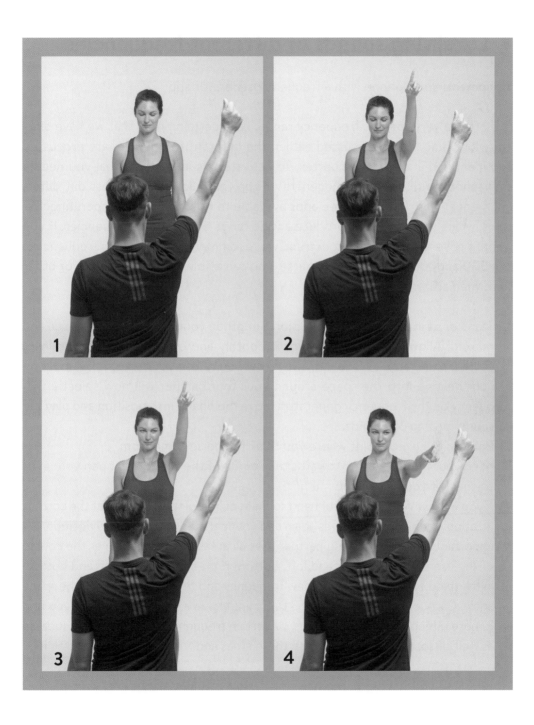

› Localising sounds of different frequencies

Equipment: Smartphone with a frequency generator app

It is often a very specific frequency range, i.e. a certain pitch, that we have difficulty localising. As we discussed earlier, the different frequencies are processed and identified in the insular cortex. To activate this important area, you need a smartphone with a frequency generator app that allows you to test out different frequencies. There are free apps available to download for all operating systems, which you can use to produce a wide range of different frequencies. If you want to cover a really broad spectrum, we recommend the following frequencies: 50, 500 and 10,000 Hertz. Of course, you can also work with a variety of other (intermediate) frequencies.

1. Stand or sit in a comfortable position. Lengthen your spine but keep it nice and relaxed. Allow your breath to flow smoothly and evenly. Have your training partner stand about 1.5 to 2 m away from you. Close your eyes, relax and tune your hearing into the space around you. Your partner will now select a frequency on the frequency generator, move their hand into position and play the sound for 2 to 3 seconds.
2. Point to the exact point where you think the noise came from.
3. Keep your finger pointed towards the source of the sound and open your eyes to check if you were right.
4. If you were wrong, move your hand so that you're pointing directly at the correct location. Then close your eyes again and your partner will pick a new position. It's important that your training partner uses all areas of the space over the course of the exercise – top right and left, bottom right and left, and top and bottom in the middle. Then switch to a new frequency and test all the areas of the space again. Carry out this exercise for 3 to 5 minutes. Are there areas where you find it more difficult to localise sounds, or certain frequencies that you can't localise as well? If so, try to focus more on these areas and frequencies in your training.

Note: Once you have got the hang of it, you can also try having your partner change the frequency from position to position. This will make the exercise even more challenging for you and will trigger even greater differentiation and integration in the insular cortex.

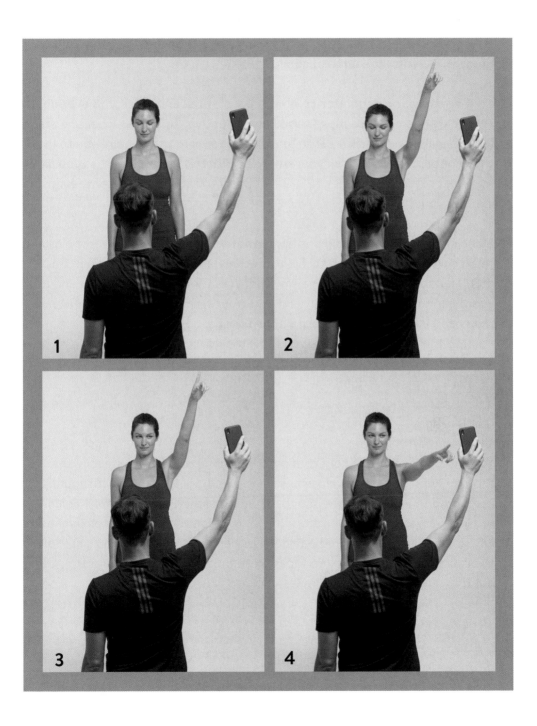

❯ Localising and tracking sounds

Equipment: A constant source of sound

Using the frequency generator to emit a constant sound gives you even more ways to make the exercise more varied and effective. As well as localising static acoustic signals, it also makes sense to include exercises that require you to localise moving sources of sound in your training. With this version, start as you did in the previous exercise on pages 228–229, but then trace the route of the moving sound with your finger.

1. Stand or sit in a comfortable position. Lengthen your spine but keep it nice and relaxed. Allow your breath to flow smoothly and evenly. Have your training partner stand about 1.5 to 2 m away from you. Close your eyes, relax and tune your hearing into the space around you. Your training partner will now move their hand into position and turn on the sound.
2. Point to the exact point where you think the noise came from.
3. Keep your finger pointed towards the source of the sound and open your eyes to check if you were right.
4. If you were wrong, move your hand so that you're pointing directly at the correct location.
5. Close your eyes again.
6. Your partner will now begin to move their hand slowly and steadily through the air. Keeping your eyes closed, trace the route of the sound with your hand. If you lose the source of the sound, let your partner know and start again. Try to use all areas of the space around you: top right and left, bottom right and left, and top and bottom in the middle. Is there an area where you can't follow the sound as well? If so, try to focus more on this area in your training. Carry out this exercise for 3 to 5 minutes.

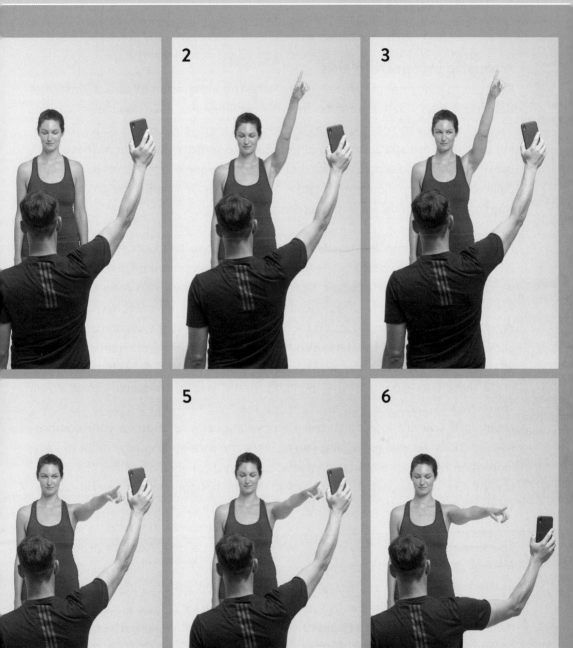

Acoustic integration aids

Because so many people are struggling with the integration of sensory information these days – largely due to the way our lifestyles have changed – various research groups and companies have dedicated themselves to this issue, developing tools that are specially designed to improve sensory integration. These tools provide a quick and simple way for you to work on your integration as part of your daily routine. They allow you to tackle this capacity in an effective and targeted way to achieve significant improvements.

For the use of acoustic signals, we recommend two products from Sound for Life. This American company specialises in the development of products for the sensory integration of acoustic signals. The first of their two main products is Forbrain®, an auditory feedback headset. This records your speech with a microphone and uses bone conduction technology to transmit the sound back to your acoustic system. Your speech is also fed back to you via the conventional route, as sound waves through the air. This forces your brain to differentiate and integrate these two variants of the sound. Forbrain® is ideal for reading texts aloud. The device is particularly effective when used with foreign language texts, for example if you are looking to learn a new language or improve your comprehension skills. As well as helping you to learn the foreign language more quickly, increasing the requirements of your acoustic system also intensifies the activation of your insular cortex. You can even use the headphones for normal conversations or phone calls – the main thing is that you're speaking.

The second product is Soundsory®, which provides a multi-sensory programme for use at home. Again, the purpose of this product is to improve integration in the insular cortex and therefore your interoceptive accuracy by increasing the requirements of the central section of your insular cortex. According to the manufacturer, it also helps to improve motor and cognitive skills. The programme comprises a series of specially developed pieces of music that are transmitted and modified using special headphones, which means your brain has to work particularly hard to integrate the modified sounds. You are then guided through a series of special movement exercises. The complete programme is designed to take 30 minutes a day for 40 days. For details on how to use these products, please refer to the manufacturer's instructions. More information can be found in the Appendix on page 302.

Categorising the exercises for acoustic mapping			
Exercise	Positive	Neutral/moderately positive	Save for later
Localising sounds (pages 226–227)			
Variation: Varying the volume (pages 226–227)			
Localising sounds of different frequencies (pages 228–229)			
Localising and tracking sounds (pages 230–231)			
Using Forbrain® (page 232)			
Using Soundsory® (page 232)			

Training recommendations for acoustic mapping

If you want to make your overall training more effective and generally increase the activation of your insular cortex, we would recommend using the exercises in this chapter as a warm-up for other elements of your training. Differentiating acoustic signals activates all sections of the insular cortex, but especially the central section, which is where sensory information is integrated. The better your brain becomes at integrating incoming signals, the more effective and sustainable the subsequent training will be. If you plan to use these exercises as a warm-up for other training or in combination with other exercises, it is sufficient to spend 3 to 5 minutes on one exercise for which you had a particularly positive assessment result.

That said, if you have found that you really struggle with localising acoustic signals – or that it has a really positive effect on you and you want to do more of it – then we recommend that you focus on these exercises for a few weeks, dedicating a whole separate training session to it. In this instance, it's best to invest 10 to 15 minutes a day, which you can of course divide into two or three shorter sessions.

Training recommendations for acoustic mapping		
Potential use	Scope and application	Effect

As the main element of the training	• Preferred combination of exercises with positive or neutral assessment results
	• 10 to 15 minutes per day in total
	• Divided into 2 or 3 sessions
		• Activates all three sections of the insular cortex
		• Improves:
		  • chronic pain
		  • interoceptive accuracy
		  • general wellbeing and fitness

As part of improving interoceptive awareness	• 1 exercise with positive assessment result • 2 to 5 minutes • 1 to 2 times per day	
Using Forbrain® and Soundsory®	Please follow the manufacturer's instructions.	
As a warm-up for other training exercises	• 1 to 2 exercises with positive assessment results • 3 to 5 minutes in total	Ideal as a warm-up for all other exercises

Eye exercises to aid relaxation

In today's digitalised world, the visual system is constantly exposed to many different stimuli. Whether it's mobile phones, computers, laptops, TV or the bombardment of visual stimuli in shopping centres and Tube stations, our visual systems are placed under extreme strain every single day. Our eyes are constantly sending visual signals to our brains, all of which have to be actively processed and integrated. This requires our brains to do a lot of work and uses up an enormous amount of energy. Your brain is constantly being stimulated and rarely has the chance to rest and recover.

Processing of visual data is one of the activities that takes place in the midbrain; more specifically, in the area that is closely connected to the sympathetic nervous system. The constant visual overload means that the sympathetic nervous system – the system responsible for performance – is always on standby, and the parasympathetic nervous system – the system responsible for rest and recovery – isn't able to work at full capacity. Therefore, if we want to reduce stress and improve the balance between the sympathetic and the parasympathetic nervous systems, we have to find ways to relieve and relax the visual system.

The significance of the ciliary muscle

The ciliary muscle – the ring of muscle that alters the shape of the lens so that we can see objects at close distance and far away – is of particular interest due to the effect it has on the autonomic nervous system. The process in which the focal length is adjusted from near to far is called 'accommodation'. When this process occurs, the ciliary muscle is activated by the third cranial nerve. The special branches of this cranial nerve are directly connected to the parasympathetic part of the nervous system and can therefore help to alleviate stress and activate the parasympathetic nervous system. In the following section, we will start by showing you two exercises that you can use as quick way to relax your visual system, including your eyes, and lower your stress level. This will be followed by an exercise designed to activate the parasympathetic nervous system by switching your gaze from near to far using the ciliary muscles. This aids regeneration and recovery.

❯ Palming and blinking

Covering your eyes is, without doubt, one of the most efficient ways to soothe your visual system and alleviate any stress in your eyes. All you need for this is your hands and 1 to 2 minutes of peace and quiet. The exercise is rounded off with a few moments of rapid blinking, which relaxes the eyes even further.

1. Sit or stand in a comfortable position. Lengthen your spine but keep it nice and relaxed. Allow your breath to flow smoothly and evenly. Start by rubbing your palms together quickly with light pressure to warm them up.
2. Close your fingers, including your thumbs, and cup your palms slightly. Place the fingers of both hands on top of each other. Make sure that your fingers are completely closed so that they block out any light.
3. Close your eyes and cover them with your warm hands. Make sure that your hands don't touch your eyes and that the entire eye area is calm and relaxed under your cupped hands. Now relax your eyes and let it get darker and darker. Focus exclusively on the increasing blackness in front of your eyes. At first, you will probably still notice little spots of light and shadow, patterns or flickers. This is normal and as you work through the exercises you'll notice them less and less until they disappear altogether. Keep going with this exercise until all you see before your eyes is a deep blackness.
4. **a+b** Then move your hands away and blink for 2 to 3 seconds as quickly as you can.

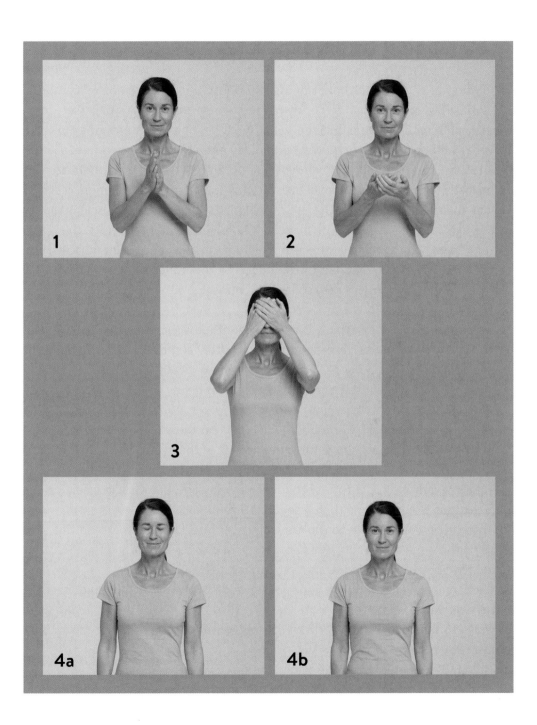

❯ Massaging the eye muscles

In addition to the bombardment of visual information, the lack of relaxation in our eyes often comes down to poorly trained eye muscles. Wearing glasses, small functional defects in the cranial nerves or your vestibular system, or simply the fact that we don't move our eyes around often enough in day-to-day life, all contribute to excessive strain and our eyes not working as well as they ought to. This often leads to tension in the small eye muscles and limits their function. Massaging the muscle insertions on the eye – the points at which the muscle attaches to the eye socket – is therefore a great way to relax and regenerate the visual system. If you look at the anatomical positioning of these important muscles, you can see that they are attached to the edges of the bones surrounding the eye socket. These insertions are easy to feel and massage with your fingers.

1. Sit or stand in a comfortable position. Lengthen your spine but keep it nice and relaxed. Allow your breath to flow smoothly and evenly. Close your eyes and feel along the bony part of your eye socket with your index finger, on the inner/rear side of the bone both above and below your eye, working your way from the inner to the outer corner of the eye. Allow your fingers to glide evenly over the edge of the bone until you feel the small bony indentations. Start the massage just above the inner corner of the eye on the upper edge of the socket. Place your fingers onto the upper inner insertion and press gently against the bone for 3 to 5 seconds. Then massage the muscle insertion for 5 seconds clockwise and then 5 seconds anti-clockwise.
2. Then move your fingers to the central upper insertion and massage this area using the same technique, pressing gently for 3 to 5 seconds and then massaging for 5 seconds clockwise and 5 seconds anti-clockwise.
3. Next, make your way to the upper outer edge of the eye socket and massage here as well.
4. Move to the lower edge, starting from the outer corner. Massage this muscle insertion too.
5. Then move along to the central lower edge of your eye socket.
6. Finally, applying light pressure in circular motions, massage the inner muscle on the lower edge of the socket.

Focus on the areas with the most tension

To achieve the best possible effects in the shortest amount of time, just focus on the eye muscles that are the most tense. To do this, use your fingers to feel the tension on each of the muscle insertions and try to notice any differences between them. Are there certain areas where you feel more tension? We often find that the muscle insertions in the inner corner – towards the nose – are a little more tense. If you have significantly more tension in some areas than others, you can work on just these areas to feel the benefits more quickly.

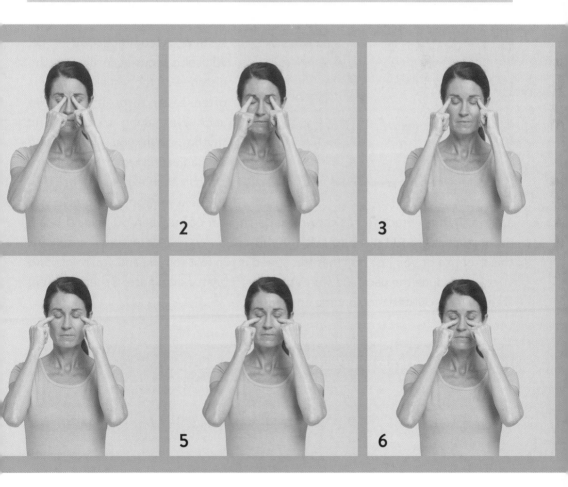

❯ Focus shifting: near and far

Equipment: Two training cards, a metronome (optional)

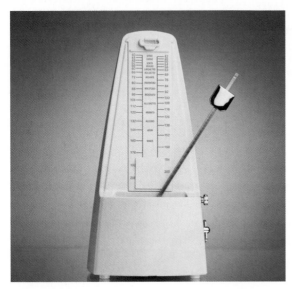

As we have already seen on page 235 in relation to the ciliary muscle, shifting our focus from near to far is a highly effective way of using the eyes to tap into the parasympathetic nervous system. Accommodation – i.e. adjusting focus according to the distance of the visual target – is often easier to do if you move your eyes along to a specific rhythm. So if you find shifting and adjusting your focus more difficult than expected, feel free to use a metronome to give you a fixed rhythm. Practice has shown that a rhythm of between 60 and 70 beats per minute is a good place to start. If you get a negative assessment result for this exercise or you just feel that this speed is too fast for you and you're getting stressed, reduce the pace and start at about 45 beats per minute. Otherwise, feel free to leave out the metronome entirely.

If focus shifting is too strenuous

Sometimes this exercise can prove to be really strenuous and intense. If this is the case for you, simply put it to one side and come back to it at a later time.

If you want to use this exercise to increase your interoceptive awareness, then – after a while – it's beneficial to use the natural rhythms from within your own body to set the pace for your focus shifting: near and far. For example, can you switch from near to far and back in time with your breath or even your heart-beat? The ability to use your body's own rhythms shows you're making major headway in your interoceptive awareness.

```
Y L E B E A S U M H
K O D S U T L O F Z
H C W A E I Q K Y R
P B V G N O A R V T
L C K O B D U T M D
A W E S P R O X N L
Z A P T I E N U R Z
V X R Y S M X J D T
S O E N R E N U H W
L B V S P D M N G H
```

```
Z M D C D B T V N G
L F E T V U M P G Y
I D X B D G R L Z T
Q C W H O P B T W U
M S L P C E V U N E
B Z F T Q S P Y O M
E B Q Z J F O W S A
W Y S Z T N Y K E U
T P F O S F O V I Y
M C W T Q E N O H I
```

For the focus shifting exercise, use one large and one small training card with the same number of rows and columns, but with different sequences of letters.

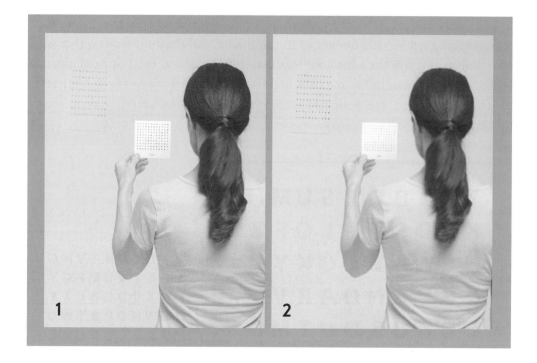

1. Sit or stand in a comfortable position. Lengthen your spine but keep it nice and relaxed. Allow your breath to flow smoothly and evenly. Hold the small training card or other visual target in front of you at eye level, at a distance of 20 to 30 cm from your eyes. Have the larger training card further away – also at eye level but attached to the wall about 2 to 5 m away. Focus on the first letter on the closest training card.

2. Then shift your focus to the first letter on the furthest training card and back to the second letter on the closest training card. Keep switching your focus between the card that's closer and the one that's further away, reading one letter after the next. It is important only to shift your focus once you have seen the letter clearly. If you're working with a metronome, adjust the speed as necessary so that you can see the letter clearly and sharply before shifting your focus again in time with the metronome. Carry out this exercise for 30 to 90 seconds.

Note: In this exercise, the crucial thing is the quality of your visual perception, rather than the speed with which you can shift your focus. Always make sure that you only shift your focus once you have a sharp view of the letter. Only the fact that you can see the letter sharply shows that your ciliary muscles have correctly adjusted the focal length. If you wear glasses or contact lenses, try to do the exercise without them, although this will be quite difficult at first. If the letter or image remains quite blurred, focus on the best possible visual acuity you can achieve. Test both variations – with and without glasses/contact lenses – by completing an assessment.

Categorising the exercises for relaxing the eyes and for the visual system			
Exercise	Positive	Neutral/ moderately positive	Save for later
Palming and blinking (pages 236–237)			
Massaging the eye muscles (pages 238–239)			
Focus shifting: near and far (pages 240–242)			
Without glasses or contact lenses			
With glasses or contact lenses			
With a metronome			
Without a metronome			
To the rhythm of your breathing			
To the rhythm of your heartbeat			

Training recommendations for relaxing the eyes and for the visual system

As a general rule, stimuli that enter the brain via the eyes are particularly powerful and can be used to quickly achieve positive effects. Most of the eye exercises we have shown you here can be slotted very easily into your daily routine. You can therefore support your parasympathetic nervous system with very little effort and reduce stress and tension. The exercises designed to relax the visual system, such as covering your eyes and blinking (pages 236–237) and massaging the eye muscles (pages 238–239), are ideal for providing quick stress relief in any stressful situation – whether that's after a long day at the office, in your coffee break, during intensive sporting activities or before public appearances and talks. You can often get the effects you want just by briefly covering your eyes or giving them a quick massage. It rarely takes any longer than 2 or 3 minutes in total. You can apply the eye relaxation techniques as many times a day as you need to.

Depending on the condition and performance of your visual system, we would recommend that you work on the accommodation exercises several times a day, for 1 or 2 minutes at a time. As with almost all the exercises in this book, focus shifting: near and far works really well in combination with other elements of interoceptive awareness training. We particularly recommend combining the exercise with wearing an abdominal belt (page 222) or respiratory training (page 123 onwards).

Training recommendations for relaxing the eyes and training the visual system		
Potential use	**Scope and application**	**Effect**

For immediate stress reduction	• Palming and blinking (pages 236–237) or massaging the eye muscles (pages 238–239)
	• 2 to 3 minutes
	• Several times a day, as required
		• Activates the parasympathetic nervous system as well as the posterior section of the insular cortex
		• Improves:
		  • recovery and regeneration
		  • stress
		  • anxiety

As part of interoceptive awareness training	• 1 to 2 minutes of focus shifting: near and far (pages 240–242)
	• 2 to 3 times per day
	• Works well combined with:
	  • wearing the abdominal belt (page 222)
	  • prolonged exhalation using the Frolov respiratory training device (page 150)
	  • prolonged exhalation using the Relaxator (pages 148–149)	

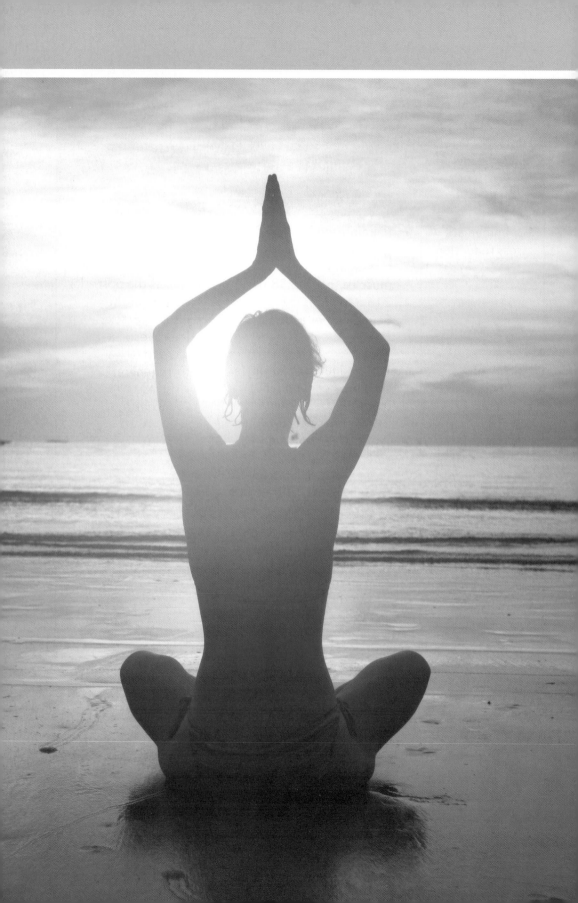

7

Body awareness
and mindfulness

Using body awareness and mindfulness exercises to activate key areas of the brain

The final topic that we would like to cover in this book is mindfulness and body awareness training. This activates all areas of your insular cortex and completes your interoceptive awareness training. Focus, concentration, attention and mindfulness are extremely important factors when it comes to improving the quality of your overall training. Simply by focusing your attention on whatever you're doing, and in particular on what's going on in your own body, you are already activating your frontal lobe and the anterior section of your insular cortex. You are already familiar with the three functional sections of the insular cortex, which we covered in the first chapter. A special feature of the anterior section of the insular cortex is that it is in constant communication with certain areas of the frontal lobe that strongly influence each other. If we look more closely at these areas of the frontal lobe, we find that exercises that focus on body awareness and mindfulness trigger high activity levels there, making them a particularly effective way of activating the anterior section of the insular cortex. By now, you'll be well aware of how important activating this area of the brain is for your health. The activity level in the anterior section of the insular cortex and in the frontal lobe, for example, has a major impact on our ability to regulate emotions. Problems with emotional regulation can range from anxiety disorders and panic attacks to depressive moods. If you practise body awareness intensively, however, this will also focus closely on the posterior section of the insular cortex, which can lead to a significant drop in stress levels, as well as alleviating digestive disorders and reducing pain.

In this chapter, we will show you a variety of body awareness and mindfulness exercises that you can easily do in the comfort of your own home. If you find that this sort of training works well for you and you notice positive effects, we would strongly encourage you to delve more deeply into this topic, beyond the exercises shown in this book. Nowadays, there is a huge selection of books, courses, programmes and apps available for mindfulness and body awareness. The range of possibilities is so extensive that we would need far more than one chapter to cover them all. We would therefore like you to see the following selection of exercises as a sort of taster – a starting point on your journey to better health and wellbeing. Body awareness and mindfulness is something that should be practised regularly – ideally every day. 10 to 20 minutes a day for four to six weeks is all you need to notice significant changes.

The difference between body awareness and mindfulness

Before we begin our body awareness and mindfulness training, we'll start by looking at the differences between the two terms. Both body awareness and mindfulness are used in various areas of the health and wellness sector as an alternative way to alleviate the complaints mentioned above. Numerous health centres, wellness clinics and other facilities offer special courses for this.

Mindfulness and body awareness are primarily about relaxing the whole body, both mentally and physically. For this book, we have chosen three exercises that you may have already come across in one form or another. These include a simplified version of Jacobson's progressive muscle relaxation technique, a body scan – a relaxation technique that reduces stress – and a mindfulness meditation that focuses on your breathing. But first let's take a closer look at the terms 'body awareness' and 'mindfulness'.

Why body awareness is so important

Body awareness exercises focus the attention on what's happening within the body, with the aim of consciously noticing and initiating certain processes. You might focus on one part of the body or on a process that takes place inside the body. A simple example of this would be the heartbeat. How does your heartbeat feel? Is your heart beating quickly or slowly? The exercises may also focus on breathing or simply noticing specific parts or areas of the body. The ultimate aim is to consciously induce changes in your physical state and initiate bodily processes by analysing, assessing and altering the information you perceive. Body awareness – using all of the senses – can be done while at rest or while moving, and is often combined with focused breathing. Body awareness exercises, including Jacobson's progressive muscle relaxation technique, can be used to address a range of complaints, including digestive disorders, pelvic floor problems, issues with blood pressure, symptoms of pain and general stress, as well as the feeling of not being at home in your own body.

The significance of mindfulness

Mindfulness is the term used to describe a type of perception in which you consciously draw your attention to the present moment – without judgement. This means that you bring your awareness to physical processes without attempting to analyse or evaluate them cognitively, i.e. by assigning conscious thoughts or emotions to them. People with excessive body awareness often struggle with mindfulness training to begin with. In spite of this – or, in fact, because of this – it is one of the most important exercises we can do. If you're someone who is highly sensitive and tuned in to what's happening in your own body and you are constantly trying to identify, interpret and evaluate these signals, you should start with the mindfulness meditation that focuses on your breathing on pages 257–258, and come back to the body awareness exercises at a later date. Mindfulness meditation is about noticing physical processes rather than trying to evaluate or alter them. Frequently and excessively listening out for what's happening in your body and trying to evaluate what you think you are noticing or feeling suggests that the insular cortex and interoceptive system aren't working as they should. In simple terms, the insular cortex is unable to adequately integrate and evaluate the information it receives, which forces the brain to try to interpret the sensory information through cognitive evaluation.

Scientific studies have shown that, particularly in the case of symptoms such as anxiety, anxiety disorders, depression and problems with emotional regulation, there is usually a disruption in the activity level of the insular cortex, which is what causes this preoccupation with what's happening inside the body. Exercises that focus on the body, such as the progressive muscle relaxation technique and the body scan, can exacerbate these symptoms. We therefore cannot stress enough that, if this applies to you, the best place to start is with mindfulness training.

Body awareness training with Jacobson's progressive muscle relaxation technique

The progressive muscle relaxation technique was developed by an American doctor called Edmund Jacobson (1888–1983). He spent 20 years researching the connection between excessive muscle tone and various physical and mental illnesses, before publishing his results for the first time in 1929, in a specialist book aimed at the medical community. Five years later, he wrote his first book for general audiences, entitled *You Must Relax*. It wasn't until 1990 that this was translated into German with the title *Entspannung als Therapie – progressive Relaxation in Theorie und Praxis* (Relaxation as therapy – progressive relaxation in theory and practice).

His research showed that the central nervous system is less active when the muscles are relaxed. This means that relaxing the muscles can also normalise our emotions and states of arousal. Being consciously aware of the body by deliberately tensing and relaxing certain muscles is therefore a very effective way to regulate the activity level of the insular cortex. When we look at the process of tensing and relaxing the muscles, as used in Jacobson's progressive muscle relaxation technique, we can see that it has numerous positive effects:

- It increases the intensity with which we feel the different areas of the body.
- It improves our perception of the position and shape of each muscle, which sends a lot of information to the insular cortex.
- Generating and controlling a strong, prolonged muscle contraction forces us to balance and adjust the autonomous functions. This, in turn, increases activity in the insular cortex.
- It slightly inhibits blood flow for a short time. This causes the blood to build up and the muscle to swell slightly, causing displacement of the fluids within the muscle.
- It alters the composition of the blood gases in the muscle because a lot of oxygen is consumed during the tension phase.

The information regarding the muscle tension, fluid displacement and altered composition of the blood gases is of course interoceptive, in that it relates to autonomous processes that are perceived and regulated in the insular cortex. By suddenly relaxing the muscle, you can clearly notice the difference between tension and relaxation. You feel the pressure subside, the blood begin to flow again and the muscle warm up and expand. This information is also transported mainly to the areas of the brain that are responsible for interoception, where it is differentiated and processed.

This small but important exercise therefore has the potential to trigger high amounts of activity in the posterior and anterior sections of the insular cortex, which has a very positive effect on interoceptive awareness. This makes muscle relaxation an especially useful tool for improving our interoceptive accuracy, reducing the symptoms of pain and chronic pain, as well as alleviating physical symptoms such as digestive disorders and balancing out fluctuations in blood pressure. The method we use in this book is a simplified version of Jacobson's progressive muscle relaxation technique.

❯ Jacobson's progressive muscle relaxation technique

Most people find this simplified version of Jacobson's muscle relaxation technique very quick and easy to learn. It therefore makes a good starting point for your body awareness training. If you do 10 minutes of conscious practice each day, you will notice an improvement in your perception of physical tension in just a few weeks.

Find yourself a space with no distractions

In order to be able to practise without distractions, it is important from the very start to create an environment in which you feel comfortable, and where you won't be disturbed or interrupted by outside noise or other people during your practice. So choose a room that feels calm and has a comfortable temperature. Switch off your mobile phone and, if necessary, dim the light. Make sure you are wearing loose, comfortable clothing. Take off your shoes and, if you plan to practise lying down, use a soft, comfortable surface to lay on, such as a blanket.

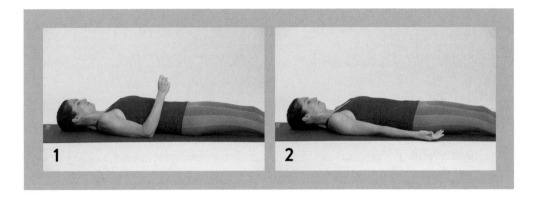

1. Lay down on a soft surface, such as a blanket, with your body loose and relaxed. Relax your arms by your sides. Allow your breath to flow smoothly and evenly. Focus your awareness on your right forearm – from the wrist up to the elbow. Hold your attention here for 2 to 3 seconds. Clench your right hand into a fist and tense your entire forearm as tightly as you possibly can. Build up the tension slowly, tightening it more and more until you have achieved the maximum possible tension in your whole forearm and hand. Pay attention to the tension and intensity for 6 to 8 seconds. During this time, let your attention wander around each part of the forearm and hand. Are you able to feel the tension equally well throughout this whole area? Are there places you can't feel it so well?

2. Abruptly release the tension. Return your attention to your forearm and hand and notice the feeling of relaxation, lightness and looseness following the tension. Notice how different your arm feels when it is relaxed, compared to when it was tensed. Now focus your attention on all parts of your forearm and hand and hold it there for a total of 30 to 60 seconds. Are all the muscles loose and relaxed? Are there areas that don't feel quite so relaxed? Notice again the difference between tension and relaxation and then repeat the exercise. Then focus your attention on the next part of your body:

   • Right forearm including hand
   • Right upper arm
   • Left forearm including hand
   • Left upper arm

- Face
- Neck
- Shoulders
- Back
- Stomach
- Right foot
- Right calf
- Right thigh
- Left foot
- Left calf
- Left thigh

You can also vary the suggested sequence if you prefer. If you feel that a certain area has particularly positive effects for you, feel free to spend a little longer there. Use the assessments in Chapter 2 from page 36 onwards to work out the sequence and length that works best for you. It's perfectly fine to start by focusing on just two or three parts of your body. If this feels good for you and you decide you would like to invest more time in it, then make your way through the whole body.

Note: During progressive muscle relaxation, it's important to ensure that you only ever tense one part of the body in isolation, and that the rest of your body stays as loose and relaxed as possible. This takes a bit of practice, but it's a really important skill to learn.

Mindfulness training

To put it simply, mindfulness is about becoming aware of whatever is happening in the present moment without judging or evaluating it. The term 'mindfulness' was coined by molecular biologist Jon Kabat-Zinn, whose research and associated MBSR programme (Mindfulness-Based Stress Reduction) in the late 1970s has shaped our understanding of the concept in the Western world. The MBSR pro-gramme is still in use all over the world today. In the following section, we will be showing you two exercises that are great for mindfulness training: the body scan and a mindfulness meditation that focuses on your breathing.

If you find that this form of practice works well for you, we would encourage you to explore other ways of expanding your practice. For example, you could try the Headspace app, which is – in our opinion – the best app on the market right now. It offers a range of basic guided meditations that are between 3 and 10 minutes long, plus lots of tips for specific subject areas.

Mindfulness training using the body scan

The body scan is an exercise that helps focus your attention on your body. It has its origins in Buddhism, where it was used as a form of meditation. The body scan as we know it today was developed by Jon Kabat-Zinn.

The body scan acts as a sort of mental examination of the body. The aim is to men-tally scan your body from your head down to your feet, searching for any tension or differences in tension. Carefully scanning and noticing the various states of tension in our muscles automatically improves our perception of our own bodies. The body scan is therefore an extremely effective way to hone our interoceptive skills. It acutely activates both the posterior and anterior sections of the insular cortex, making it ideal for alleviating chronic pain or increasing the effectiveness of pelvic floor training. Furthermore, due to its effect on the anterior section of the insular cortex, it is also a great exercise for people who struggle with anxiety, react very emotionally to stress or experience intense mood swings.

We're giving you quite an abridged version of the body scan here. It's only intended to give you an introduction to the technique. If you want a more in-depth look at the body scan or the MBSR method, please refer to the recommended reading in the Appendix from page 307 onwards.

› Body scan

The body scan is an easy way to identify physical tension and – in the best-case scenario – to relieve it. It works really well for those who often feel stressed or generally find it difficult to sense what's happening in their own bodies.

Lie down on your back and relax. Lengthen your spine but keep it nice and relaxed. Allow your breath to flow smoothly and evenly. Now imagine you're scanning your body from head to toe, inch by inch, from top to bottom. Start at the head, noticing your face, head and neck. Do you feel any differences between the right and left sides of your face, the right and left sides of your skull or in your neck muscles? Is there tension anywhere? Spend a little time noticing this tension and try to resolve it simply by asking yourself, in your mind, to let it go. Using the same method, scan your shoulders, chest, arms, torso, legs and feet for any tense spots and, if there are any, use your mind to gently guide the tension out of your body.

It takes time and practice to get the hang of scanning each individual part of your body, noticing each part and allowing yourself to release the tension. But you

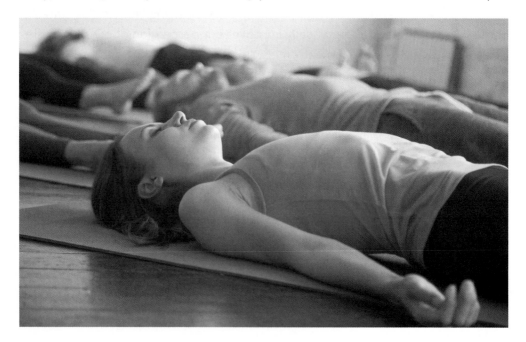

will see that it's easier than it first seems. The important thing is that you start learning to notice your body and any tension you're holding onto – and to let it go. Scan the body either in its entirety or in sections for 5 to 10 minutes each day.

Mindfulness meditation

Mindfulness training often includes mindfulness meditation, which also has its roots in the Buddhist tradition. Mindfulness, as we understand it in this book, is a meditative, focused yet relaxed process of perceiving, in which the focus is on whatever it is that we perceive. The most important thing to remember with mindfulness meditation is not to evaluate what you perceive. It is all about just acknowledging and accepting what you notice as it is now.

For example, if we used mindfulness meditation to focus on our breathing, we would notice how our breath feels as it flows in and out, without trying to analyse other aspects such as how much air is coming in through the nose, how deep the breath is or when the flow of breath changes and how.

In the following, we will show you an example of a mindfulness meditation based on a guided meditation borrowed from the mindful.org website. This website offers a range of meditations and exercises, as well as lots of interesting background information about the practice of mindfulness.

❯ Mindfulness meditation focusing on breathing

A good place to start with mindfulness meditation is to use your breathing as the focus of your attention. Aside from the effect it has on your health, your breathing makes the ideal focus because it is a constant process, and as such can be focused on in almost any place and at any time. Pay attention to the flow of breath during this exercise and notice what happens. Over the course of the exercise, you will definitely find that your attention wanders a few times as you get distracted by different thoughts, emotions or noises. This is not a problem. Wherever your attention wanders, simply guide it gently back to the present with your next breath.

1. Find a space where you feel at ease. Find something comfortable to sit on that also allows you to keep your posture stable.
2. Before you start, have a little think about what your legs are doing. If you're sitting on a cushion, you may find it comfortable to cross your legs in front of you. If you're sitting on a chair, place your feet in a relaxed position on the floor.
3. Sit up straight, but with your upper body nice and relaxed. Your spine has a natural curve, so don't be tempted to try and straighten it out too much.
4. Now have a think about what your arms are doing. Hold them out in front of you and allow your palms to rest on your legs, wherever feels most natural to you.
5. Relax your gaze. Lower your chin and eyes a little. It's up to you whether or not you close your eyes – either way is fine. If you keep them open, simply allow your gaze to settle in front of you without focusing on anything.
6. Notice your breath. Focus your attention on the physical sensation of the breath: notice how it feels as it flows in and out through your nose or mouth. Turn your attention to the movement of your stomach or rib cage. Feel how they move with each breath you take.
7. Notice if your attention moves away from your breath and your thoughts begin to wander. This is completely normal. Simply bring your attention back to your breathing.
8. Be kind to yourself and your wandering mind. Rather than trying to fight against your thoughts, simply acknowledge them, without responding to them. Continue to sit in this relaxed state and bring your focus back to your breathing, without any expectations or judgement.
9. When you feel ready, gently lift your head. If your eyes are closed, open them. Take a moment to listen to any sounds around you. Notice how your body feels. Notice any thoughts or feelings you have and bring the exercise to a close by taking a deep breath in and out.

Categorising the body awareness and mindfulness exercises			
Exercise	Positive	Neutral/moderately positive	Save for later
Jacobson's progressive muscle relaxation technique (pages 252–254)			
Body scan (pages 256–257)			
Mindfulness exercise focusing on breathing (pages 257–258)			

Use the assessments

We recommend using a mobility assessment (pages 36–39) or pain level assessment (pages 40–41) to test how effective the body awareness and mindfulness exercises are for you before you start your training.

Training recommendations for body awareness and mindfulness

There are two ways in which you can use body awareness and mindfulness training. One option is to focus on it as the main part of your training for a few weeks. As mentioned in the introduction, we would recommend practising these exercises for 10 to 20 minutes a day over the course of six to eight weeks in order to achieve a significant change in the activity level of the insular cortex and to improve specific symptoms.

Mindfulness meditation is especially recommended for anyone who struggles with emotional regulation. If you suffer from anxiety disorders, depression, stress, eating disorders, addictive tendencies or similar, doing this training for several weeks can be really helpful. We would like to reiterate here that these exercises are about supporting you to improve your interoceptive awareness and helping you to regulate the activity levels in important parts of your brain.

If you want to improve your body awareness and alleviate physical symptoms, the simplified version of Jacobson's progressive muscle relaxation technique works particularly well, as does the body scan. Of the two, the body scan includes more aspects of mindfulness and, as already mentioned, works really well for those who struggle with mood swings and stress.

You can also combine the body awareness and mindfulness exercises with some of the other training elements introduced in this book. For example, you could do a quick 2 or 3-minute body scan or a short mindfulness meditation after your breathing or pelvic floor exercises.

Training recommendations for body awareness and mindfulness		
Potential use	**Scope and application**	**Effect**

As the main element of the training	• 1 exercise with positive assessment result
	   • Progressive muscle relaxation (pages 252–254)
	   • Body scan (pages 256–257)
	   • Mindfulness meditation (pages 257–258)
	 • 10 to 20 minutes each day
	 • Practise regularly for 6 to 8 weeks
		Progressive muscle relaxation
		 • Activates the posterior section of the insular cortex
		 • Improves:
		   • chronic pain
		   • overall stress level
		   • physical problems such as digestive disorders and blood pressure problems
		 Body scan
		 • Activates the posterior and anterior sections of the insular cortex

Training recommendations for body awareness and mindfulness		
Potential use	**Scope and application**	**Effect**

As part of interoceptive awareness training	• 2 to 3 times per day
	• 1 to 2 minutes spread across the day
		• Improves:
		  • chronic pain
		  • pelvic floor problems
		Mindfulness training
		• Activates the anterior section of the insular cortex
		• Improves:
		  • anxiety
		  • depressive moods
		  • emotional regulation
		  • digestive disorders

In combination with other exercises	• Body scan or mindfulness meditation after the breathing or pelvic floor exercises • 2 to 3 minutes	• Also activates the anterior section of the insular cortex • Improves the overall effectiveness of the training

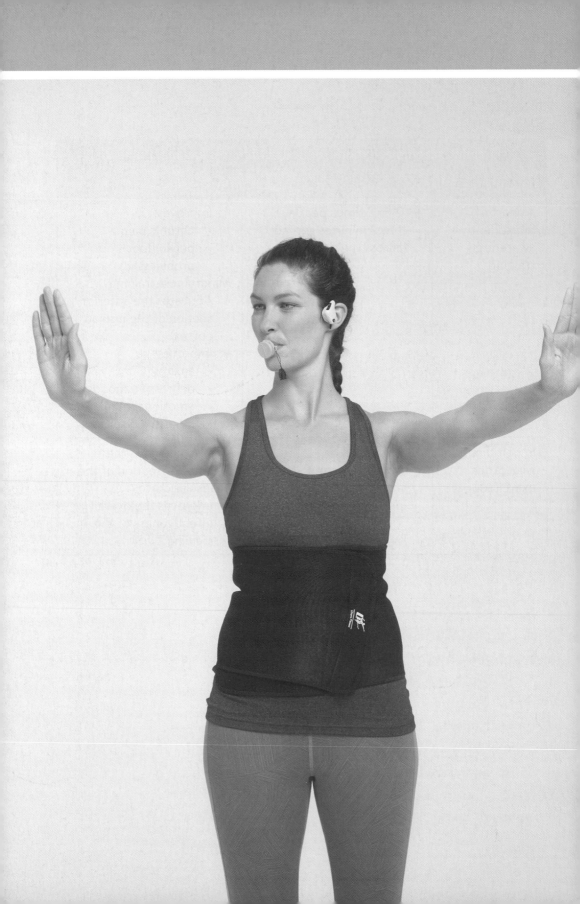

8

Specific training plans to improve your health issues

The art of selecting effective combinations for maximum success

If you've made it this far, you should already have trained the individual areas of your interoceptive awareness such as your tongue, throat or pelvic floor and will by now be noticing significant improvements. You may even have put together your own daily training plan to improve your overall interoceptive awareness, using the exercises that gave you particularly good assessment results. That's great, because this basic training is extremely important! You may even have gone so far as to select the exercises relating to your specific symptoms from the tables, and perhaps you've already made great progress towards achieving your personal goals. The aim of this chapter is to build on your progress up to this point and to give you further tools to help you achieve your personal health goals even more quickly and sustainably.

At the end of the chapter, we will give you guidance on how to address your specific symptoms and problems as effectively as possible by combining selected exercises. These combinations are specifically designed to improve the most common manifestations of poor interoceptive awareness and dysfunctions of the insular cortex. For this chapter, we have selected five categories for which we will provide you with targeted training plans:

- Category 1: Improving general health levels, reducing stress and increasing fitness
- Category 2: Reducing chronic pain
- Category 3: Improving emotional regulation
- Category 4: Alleviating digestive disorders
- Category 5: Minimising pelvic floor problems

The combinations of exercises we have selected are designed to activate the areas of the insular cortex that are involved in regulating the autonomous functions related to the symptoms you are experiencing. For example, for those living with chronic pain, it is important to activate the posterior section of the insular cortex in particular, as this is where the intensity of pain is assessed and it is also part of the neural network that determines the pain pattern. In contrast, activating the anterior section of the insular cortex is more important for those who struggle with emotional regulation. That said, it's not just the area of the insular cortex that's important, but also the type of information that the brain needs more of in order to improve the specific symptoms.

Although this chapter is very important in helping you to achieve your personal health goals, it should not encourage you to neglect the work you are doing on the individual aspects of your interoceptive awareness, such as breathing exercises, tongue training or working on the basic parameters. On the contrary, the better these individual systems work and the better the quality of the information sent to the insular cortex from these areas, the more effective these combinations of exercises will be for improving your health.

Performing several exercises at the same time

As you've worked through the individual chapters, you will already have seen how important it is to warm up the different brain areas and neurological structures involved in processing information. This helps us to achieve the effects we're looking for more quickly and more easily, and makes the overall training better and more efficient. Now let's take this one step further. By bringing in multiple stimuli, we can increase the ability of the brain and the nervous system to adapt to the training. There are two ways to achieve this using the exercise combinations introduced in this chapter:

1. **Performing the exercises in quick succession:** This approach involves using different stimuli, one after the other. It is particularly suitable for people who find it difficult to multi-task. The important thing here is to ensure that each exercise is carried out in quick succession, with a break of no longer than 15 seconds between each one.
2. **Performing the exercises simultaneously:** An example of this approach would be to combine wearing the abdominal belt (page 222) with saccades (page 56) in order to activate the frontal lobe, while also using the Relaxator for prolonged exhalation (pages 148–149). Practice has shown that this approach is often more effective than performing the exercises one after the other. It's ideal for people who have little difficulty focusing on and coordinating several physical processes at once.

However, both approaches increase the amount and the variety of stimulation in specific areas of the brain, resulting in more acute activation than each stimulus would be able to achieve individually. The increased intensity of the activation enables the brain to make neuroplastic changes more quickly and sustainably.

As well as increasing the number of stimuli, there is another principle that can be used to boost the effect of your training. As you already know, the intensity and strength of a stimulus also determines its effect on the nervous system. In other words: the stronger the stimulus, the greater the adjustment. Practice has shown that stimuli from sensory organs that are closer to the brain, such as the tongue, eyes and vestibular system, generally effect more intense stimulation than areas that are further away from the brain. We have therefore included more of these types of exercises in this chapter. You could think of them as a sort of catalyst for your training.

Improving integration through targeted pre-activation

Remember: All the information that is received by the insular cortex has to be integrated there. If the insular cortex isn't functioning properly, this has negative consequences for the entire process. The activity level of this area of the brain, which is responsible for integration, is therefore extremely important. The information that makes it to the insular cortex is integrated in the central section. This also contains processing centres for taste and smell. We like to use olfactory and gustatory stimuli, not only due to the proximity of these sensory organs to the brain, but also because they activate the integration centre in the central section of the insular cortex. This gives us a head start when it comes to improving the brain's capacity for integrating and processing incoming sensory information.

Warm-up exercises

The smell and taste exercises that you covered in Chapter 3 on pages 90 to 97 can each be used as a short warm-up before you start the main exercise combinations. It also makes sense to get started with a tongue exercise that gave you a positive assessment result – unless there's already a tongue exercise included in the combination. Remember: The tongue has a number of positive effects on your health. Think of it as your secret weapon for neuroplasticity and healing! Feel free to have another read through the information about the tongue in Chapter 5, from page 183 onwards.

Using the assessments for the exercise combinations

Don't forget that you already have a very important tool to help you get the best out of your training – the assessments, which can be found in Chapter 2, from page 31 onwards. These can also be used for combinations of exercises. For some people, a combination that uses four different stimuli might work perfectly, while for others that could be too many or too few. Regularly test the effectiveness of your training and adapt it to your specific needs and the current condition of your nervous system. Since this chapter is about targeting specific symptoms, we would advise checking repeatedly whether the training is having an effect on the symptom you're focusing on – ideally, as soon as you've finished. Ask yourself: Has the pain subsided? Is there any difference in your sense of wellbeing, stress level, digestion or emotional state? Of course, for certain regulation processes, this takes a little time. That's why you need to regularly take a step back and use the assessments to monitor how you're doing and what effects the training is having.

Don't want to use the assessments?

It's not unusual, especially when we're going through particularly stressful periods in our lives, to feel uneasy about the idea of 'being tested'. If you would prefer not to do the tests, simply choose a combination of exercises that you can coordinate well and that you feel comfortable with. By 'comfortable', we don't necessarily mean that you should find the combination easy, but rather that you should feel safe and confident while doing it. Don't forget – this is exercise after all, and it's okay if it's a bit demanding.

Category 1: Improving general health, reducing stress and increasing physical fitness

For anyone seeking to generally improve their health, reduce their stress levels and feel as fit as possible, it's important to start by combining lots of exercises that activate the posterior section of the insular cortex. To help you identify these, we have included a note in the training recommendation tables at the end of each chapter, showing you which exercises address which area of the insular cortex.

The main thing here is to include a variety of breathing and vestibular exercises in your combinations, as these activate the posterior section of the insular cortex particularly intensively. To get the best results with the least amount of effort, we recommend that you use certain tools and training aids to provide stimulation for you. For example, simply wearing an abdominal belt (page 222) applies pressure that causes various interoceptive signals to be transmitted to the insular cortex over a long period – with many benefits. We also like to use 'bone conduction headphones'.

Bone conduction headphones – the perfect way to support your vestibular system

The information from the vestibular system sends a vast number of signals to the insular cortex, where they are integrated and linked to other sensory information. The vestibular system is therefore one of the most important systems for laying the foundations on which to improve your interoceptive awareness, as well as the activity levels and processes in the insular cortex. This is in fact why vestibular training is one of the central and most crucial aspects of this book. We would now like to introduce you to a very efficient way of activating this important system. As well as the exercises already mentioned, which involve active stimulation, it is also possible to tap into a large part of the vestibular system through passive stimulation. This involves transmitting acoustic signals to the vestibular organs via the cranial bones in which the organs are embedded.

The macular organs – the utricle and saccule – are particularly sensitive to a certain frequency range. We can therefore use the bone conduction headphones to directly stimulate various components of the macular organs. The bone conduction headphones don't sit inside or over your ears like conventional headphones, but sit directly on the temporal bone – the part of the skull just in front of the concha. From here, the frequencies are transmitted into the inner ear through the bone. This is where the acoustic and sensory perception of the vibration occurs – i.e. you hear and feel the sound. Rehabilitation of vestibular disorders typically involves using very specific frequencies to activate both macular organs. A frequency range of around 100 Hz (Hertz) is used to stimulate the utricle, and a range of around 500 Hz to stimulate the saccule. Such precise activation is only possible with medical equipment. Practice has shown that frequencies above and below each of these values also have a positive effect on the health and function of the vestibular organs. This is really useful to know if we want to get the best results from our interoceptive awareness and vestibular training. It's definitely worth investing in a pair of bone conduction headphones. You will also need a frequency generator so that you can send the right frequencies to the headphones. There are various apps available for each operating system. More information can be found in the Appendix on page 304.

The use of bone conduction headphones is, without doubt, the easiest way to provide effective and long-lasting stimulation to your vestibular system throughout the day, resulting in significant improvements. If the function of your vestibular system is impaired and you find the active vestibular exercises difficult, then the bone conduction headphones are the ideal solution for you. Remember: The longer and more intensively you train, the more sustainable will be the effects of the training.

❯ Passive stimulation of the vestibular system using bone conduction headphones

Equipment: Bone conduction headphones and smartphone with frequency generator

1. Sit or stand in a comfortable position. Lengthen your spine but keep it nice and relaxed. Allow your breath to flow smoothly and evenly. Place the bone conduction headphones on your head so that the speakers are positioned on the bone right in front of the concha. Connect the bone conduction headphones – via Bluetooth or using the cable provided – to the smartphone that has the frequency generator app installed on it. Choose an assessment from the 'mobility' category (Chapter 2, page 36 onwards) and carry it out. Make a note of your range of movement and how tense you feel.
2. Open the app on your phone and set the frequency generator to emit sound to both headphones. Select a frequency of 100 Hz and a speed of between 40 and 60 bpm (beats per minute). You should then be able to hear and feel a low

tone or vibration at the selected speed. Leave this frequency to work for 30 to 40 seconds and then repeat your assessment.

3. Make a note of the result and then switch to a frequency range of 500 Hz. Leave this frequency to work for 30 to 40 seconds and then repeat the assessment again. Compare the results of both frequencies with one another. When using the bone conduction headphones with the following combinations, pick the frequency that gave you the best assessment result.

Note: Test the effects of various frequencies in between. What results do you get with 150 Hz or 450 Hz, for example? At the start, you will likely find that there are particular frequency ranges that you respond best to. In the long term, however, you should work with a variety of different frequencies to make your training different every time, forcing your brain and nervous system to adapt to different stimuli.

Tip: Because the bone conduction headphones are so simple to use and yet extremely effective, you should try combining this stimulus with exercises that focus on other aspects of your interoceptive awareness. This is the perfect way to supplement your vestibular training (Chapter 3, page 64 onwards). We generally recommend that you incorporate use of the bone conduction headphones into as many aspects of your training as possible. All you have to do is select the frequency that suits you, get the headphones into the correct position and start the app.

Possible combinations

Over the next few pages, we will be showing you a variety of highly effective example combinations that should help you to achieve your training goals effectively, with lasting results. Use the suggested combinations as a basis for creating your own combinations for Category 1. However, always use the assessments to test how effective a combination is and don't overwhelm yourself. Try to stick to a training or application time of around 20 minutes a day in order to comply with the principles of neuroplasticity and to bring about long-term change.

› Combination 1　　Duration: 3 to 4 minutes

Equipment: Abdominal belt, Z-Vibe, small fragrance bottles

Exercise	Page
Wearing an abdominal belt	222
Sensory stimulus of the auricular branch	107
Tongue circles	191
Differentiating and identifying smells	92–93

Preparation: Start by putting the abdominal belt on. It should close tightly but still sit comfortably around your middle. Hold the Z-Vibe in one hand and a fragrance bottle in the other.

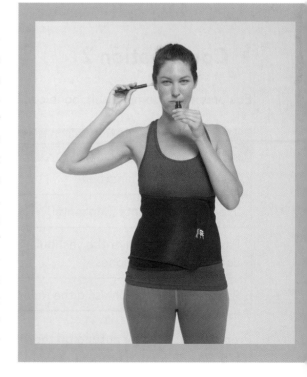

Stand up straight with your feet shoulder-width apart, keeping your spine nice and relaxed. Start to vibrate the skin on the inside of your right concha, while simultaneously circling your tongue and holding the fragrance bottle under your nose with your left hand, breathing in the smell. Make sure that you stay loose and relaxed. Throughout the exercise, keep taking the fragrance bottle away from your nose, letting your olfactory receptors relax for a moment. You will also need to take an occasional short break from circling your tongue. Feel free to repeat this combination three to five times a day.

Notes

- This combination should take at least 3 to 4 minutes. You can of course continue for longer if you wish. However, make sure that you feel comfortable at all times and, for example, that the vibration on your ear doesn't begin to feel unpleasant or stressful. It's sufficient to incorporate 1 or 2 minutes of sensory stimulus of the auricular branch into this combination. Change the fragrance regularly to keep the training varied and interesting.
- If you find it difficult to coordinate this combination of exercises, try leaving out either the fragrance element or the tongue circles, doing this for 1 or 2 minutes beforehand instead. The rest of the combination remains unchanged and you can simply carry on with it as described.

Tip: With this combination, you can also hold your breath once or twice while circling your tongue, to introduce an element of air hunger without having to change anything about the setting. Of course, this is only possible while you're taking a little break from smelling the fragrance.

❯ Combination 2   Duration: 2 to 4 minutes

Equipment: Abdominal belt, bone conduction headphones and app, Relaxator

Exercise	Page
Wearing an abdominal belt	222
'No-no' movements (horizontal)	66–67
Passive stimulation of the vestibular system using bone conduction headphones	269–270
Prolonged exhalation using the Relaxator	148–149

Preparation: Start by putting on the abdominal belt nice and tightly, and placing the bone conduction headphones into the right position on your temporal bones.

Choose a frequency for which you had a positive assessment result. Adjust the
audio on the app to a rhythm that you can also use for your head movements.

a+b: Stand upright with your feet shoulder-width apart and your spine lengthened but relaxed. Place the Relaxator loosely between your lips. Lift your
arms to about eye level and make sure that they're parallel to one another.
Focus your attention on your breathing. Take a deep breath in through your
nose, and a long breath out through the Relaxator. Now begin the 'no-no'
movements, moving your head alternately towards your right then left hand.
It's important to stay cool and relaxed despite the multitude of stimuli, and
to continue the breathing exercise while moving your head. This combination should take a total of 2 to 4 minutes and be repeated three to four
times a day.

Notes
- There's no doubt that, at first, it's difficult to coordinate everything and keep
all the exercises going at the same time. The 'no-no' movements, in particular,
are very challenging to keep up for a long time. However, you will gradually get

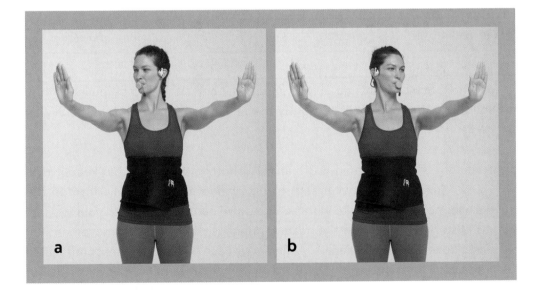

the hang of it. You can take a short break at any time and then continue the training. This won't have any impact on its effectiveness.

• Feel free to adjust the speed of the head movements to the rhythm of the selected frequency range. We recommend a speed of around 40 to 60 bpm, which is about the right amount of time to move your head from right to left and back again in one beat. If you only plan to do one movement per beat, you can use a speed of 80 to 120 bpm. So you would move your head to the right with one beat and to the left with the next, and so on. Alternatively, you can also use a continuous tone and move your head at your own speed without using a specific number of beats.

❯ Combination 3 a   Duration: 3 to 4 minutes

Equipment: Abdominal belt, Z-Vibe

Exercise	Page
Wearing an abdominal belt	222
Vibrating the front teeth	110
'Yes-yes' movements (vertical)	70–71

Preparation: Start by putting on the abdominal belt. It should be pulled tightly around the stomach, but not so tightly that it's uncomfortable. Hold the Z-Vibe in one hand.

a+b: Stand with your feet hip-width apart. Lengthen your spine but keep it nice and relaxed. Allow your breath to flow smoothly and evenly. Turn on the Z-Vibe so that it starts to vibrate. Bite down gently onto it with your incisors and start to accelerate the head continuously in a 'yes-yes' movement, up and down and back up again. Adjust your pace so that you feel comfortable and you can still control your head movements. Carry out this combination for a total of 3 to 4 minutes at a time, and repeat three to four times per day.

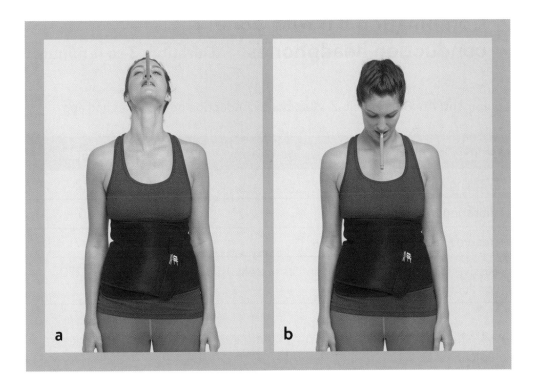

a   b

Note: Feel free to take a break in between – head movements are particularly difficult to perform continuously for a long time. You will gradually get better at it and will be able to do it for longer. Make sure that you feel comfortable at all times and that the vibration on your teeth doesn't begin to feel unpleasant or cause you stress. Several bursts of dental vibration for 20 seconds at a time is plenty for this combination.

Tip: You can also use prolonged exhalation using the Relaxator (pages 148–149) instead of the dental vibration.

❯ Combination 3 b with bone conduction headphones Duration: 3 to 4 minutes

Equipment: Abdominal belt, Z-Vibe, bone conduction headphones and app

Exercise	Page
Wearing an abdominal belt	222
Vibrating the front teeth	110
'Yes-yes' movements (vertical)	70–71
Passive stimulation of the vestibular system using bone conduction headphones	269–270

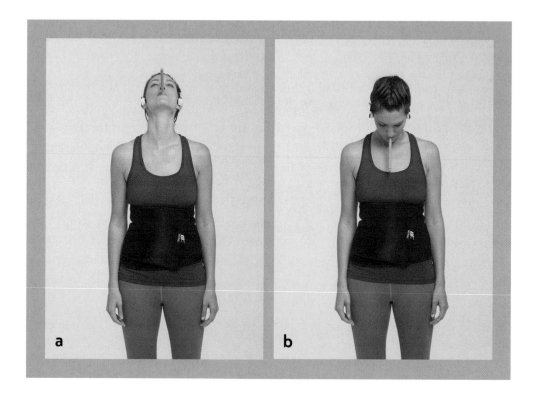

a b

Preparation: Start by putting on the abdominal belt. It should be pulled tightly around the stomach, but not so tightly that it's uncomfortable. Place the bone conduction headphones into the right position on your temporal bones and select a frequency for which you had a positive assessment result. Adjust the audio on the app to a rhythm that you can also use for your head movements. Hold the Z-Vibe in one hand.

a+b: For this combination, use the method as described for Combination 3 a on pages 274–275, but also wear the bone conduction headphones. Continue this combination of exercises for a total of 3 to 4 minutes at a time, and repeat three to five times throughout the day.

Note: Again, feel free to adjust the speed of your head movements to the rhythm of the selected frequency range. We recommend a speed of around 40 to 60 bpm, which is about the right amount of time to move your head down and up and back down again in one beat. If you only plan to do one movement per beat, use a speed of 80 to 120 bpm. So you would move your head down with one beat and up with the next beat, and so on. Alternatively, you can use a continuous tone and move your head at your own speed.

❯ Combination 4 a   Duration: 3 to 4 minutes

Equipment: Abdominal belt, Z-Vibe

Exercise	Page
Wearing an abdominal belt	222
'No-no' movements (horizontal)	66–67
Sensory stimulus of the auricular branch	107
Tongue side to side	192

Preparation: Start by putting on the abdominal belt. It should be pulled tightly around the stomach, but not so tightly that it's uncomfortable. Hold the Z-Vibe in one hand.

a+b: Stand with your feet hip-width apart. Lengthen your spine but keep it nice and relaxed. Allow your breath to flow smoothly and evenly. Begin the 'no-no' movements, moving your head rapidly from right to left. Now start flicking your tongue from side to side in time with your head movements, pushing your tongue into your left cheek as you move your head to the left, and into your right cheek as you move your head to the right. If you can, you could also try vibrating the right concha. Carry out this combination of exercises for 3 to 4 minutes at a time. You can repeat this three to five times per day.

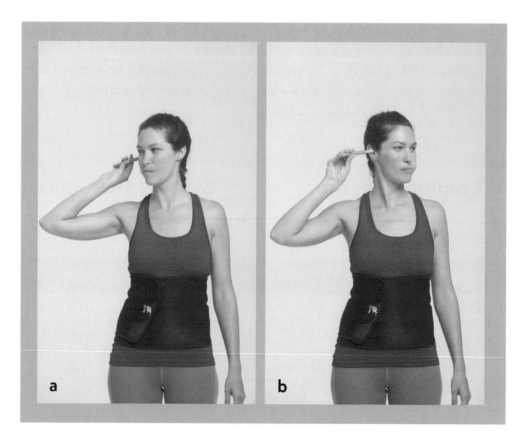

Note: If you prefer, it's perfectly fine to vibrate the ear separately for 1 to 2 minutes beforehand and then combine the rest of the exercises. Feel free to take a break in between – both the head movements and the tongue exercises can be difficult to keep up for a long time. That said, you will gradually get better at it and will be able to do it for longer.

› Combination 4 b with bone conduction headphones   Duration: 3 to 4 minutes

Equipment: Abdominal belt, bone conduction headphones and app, Z-Vibe

Exercise	Page
Wearing an abdominal belt	222
'No-no' movements (horizontal)	66–67
Passive stimulation of the vestibular system using bone conduction headphones	269–270
Sensory stimulus of the auricular branch	107
Tongue side to side	192

Preparation: Start by putting on the abdominal belt. It should be pulled tightly around the stomach, but not so tightly that it's uncomfortable. Place the bone conduction headphones into the right position on your temporal bones and select a frequency for which you had a positive assessment result. Adjust the audio on the app to a rhythm that you can also use for your head movements. Hold the Z-Vibe in one hand.

a+b: For this combination of exercises, use the method as described for Combination 4 a on pages 277–278, but also wear the bone conduction headphones. Carry out this combination for 3 to 4 minutes at a time. You can repeat this three to five times per day.

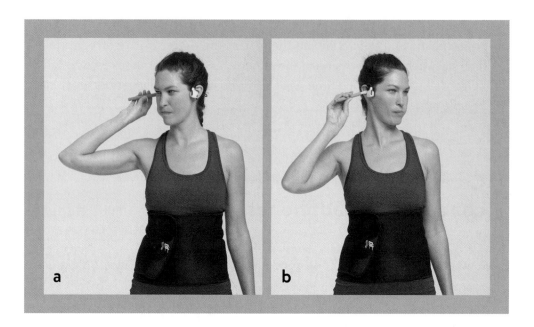

Note: Feel free to take a few short breaks if the continuous head movements cause you difficulty. You will gradually get better at it and will be able to do it for longer. You can also adjust the speed of your head movements to the rhythm of the selected frequency range. For this, we recommend a speed of around 40 to 60 or 80 to 120 bpm. Alternatively, you can use a continuous tone.

Vary the vestibular exercises

For combinations 2, 3 and 4, you can pick and choose between the seven basic vestibular exercises on pages 66 to 85 to keep the training varied. Your options here are 'no-no' movements (pages 66–67), Variation 1: 'No-no' movements with eyes closed (pages 67–68), Variation 2: 'No-no' movements with a clear visual target (pages 68–69), 'yes-yes' movements (pages 70–71), Variation 1: 'Yes-yes' movements with eyes closed (pages 71–72), Variation 2: 'Yes-yes' movements with a clear visual target (pages 72–73) and lateral head tilts (page 74). Choose an exercise for which you had a positive or neutral assessment result.

› Combination 5

Duration: 3 to 4 minutes

Equipment: Abdominal belt, Frolov respiratory training device, two training cards

Exercise	Page
Wearing an abdominal belt	222
Exhalation using the Frolov respiratory training device	150
Focus shifting: near and far	240–242

Preparation: Start by putting on the abdominal belt. It should be pulled tightly around the stomach, but not so tightly that it's uncomfortable. Follow the manufacturer's instructions to fill the Frolov respiratory training device with water. Hold the Frolov device in one hand and the small near/far training card in the other. Attach the large near/far training card to the wall in front of you at a distance of 2 to 5 m away.

a+b: Stand with your feet hip-width apart. Lengthen your spine but keep it nice and relaxed. Start with the breathing exercise using the Frolov respiratory training device. Focus on noticing your breath for three to four inhalations and exhalations. Now begin to shift your focus from near to far. Carry out this combination for 3 to 4 minutes at a time. You can repeat this exercise combination three to five times per day.

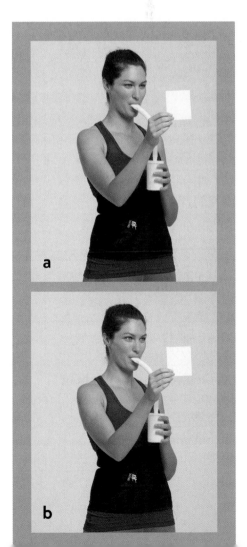

Note: Make sure that you stay calm and relaxed throughout. Remember, it will take time to get used to each new combination of exercises. Feel free to take a break from time to time, if you need to.

Tip: Instead of focus shifting: near and far you are welcome to do the saccades or horizontal eye movements (page 56) instead. This triggers an even stronger activation of the frontal lobe, whereas the focus shifting: near and far has a more intense impact on your parasympathetic nervous system. You can also warm up for this combination by doing the 'differentiating and identifying smells' exercise (pages 92–93) for 20 to 30 seconds.

Categorising the combinations for improving health, reducing stress and increasing fitness levels			
Combination	Positive	Neutral/moderately positive	Save for later
Combination 1 (pages 271–272)			
Combination 2 (pages 272–274)			
Combination 3 a (pages 274–275)			
Combination 3 b with bone conduction headphones (pages 276–277)			
Combination 4 a (pages 277–279)			
Combination 4 b with bone conduction headphones (pages 279–280)			
Combination 5 (pages 281–282)			

Training recommendations for improving general health, reducing stress and increasing physical fitness

We recommend that you continue your interoceptive awareness training to improve your health, reduce stress and increase your fitness level for a period of six to eight weeks. You should spend at least 20 minutes on your training per day. For this, use the combinations for which you had positive or neutral assessment results. Vary your training slightly from week to week to keep giving your brain new challenges. There are several ways in which you can do this: choose a different combination of exercises each time, change the speed or breathing resistance, or choose a different smell. Be creative and challenge your brain's adaptability!

Category 2: Chronic pain

If you suffer from chronic pain, it usually takes a little longer to change the underlying neural connections. The longer you've been experiencing the symptoms, the more work it usually takes to get the neural networks responsible for experiencing pain back on the right track. You have to be willing to invest a lot of time, patience and determination, but rest assured that your commitment will pay off! The main way to combat chronic pain is to improve the overall activation of the posterior section of the insular cortex. We will also be incorporating local stimulation of the specific areas of pain. Irrespective of your pain level, you're sure to notice improvements in other areas in no time at all, such as feeling more relaxed, digesting your food better, or improved regeneration. These are all signs that your system is beginning to restructure and rearrange itself. Enjoy these changes! They show that you're going in the right direction.

Local stimulation of the skin using light touch or vibration

For this particular goal, there is another way in which you can achieve positive changes with little effort, simply by lightly touching or vibrating the skin. Both of these stimuli have several positive effects that we can benefit from. Firstly, they stimulate the free nerve endings of the C fibres, which send information to the exact area of the insular cortex that is responsible for providing an adequate assessment of the intensity of pain. Secondly, this information is used to obtain a larger quantity of more differentiated information from the painful area. By stimulating the skin around the painful area, the thalamus in particular – the specific area of the brain that is heavily involved in the development of pain patterns – receives new and 'pain-free' information from the area, forcing it to reclassify and reassess the entire situation. This information effectively forces the thalamus to begin the whole process of differentiation from scratch, which often leads to rapid improvement of the pain patterns. The important thing here is that you test the immediate effects of the stimulation. Because persistent pain can cause highly sensitive responses, start by testing the effects of the exercise on the painful area itself. If this turns out to be uncomfortable or causes additional pain, then test the skin around the painful area.

Testing your ability to hold your breath is a particularly informative way of evaluating how effective it is for you to use gentle touch or vibration to stimulate your skin. You should therefore test how easy or difficult you find it to hold your breath (pages 155–156) both before and after the exercise. If you see an improvement, this exercise clearly works well for you and you can incorporate it into your exercise combinations.

❯ Stimulating the skin using light touch

Equipment: A thin cloth or handkerchief

1. Stand or sit in a comfortable position. Lengthen your spine but keep it nice and relaxed. Allow your breath to flow smoothly and evenly. Take a thin cloth and use it to touch the skin in the painful area. Stroke the cloth slowly and gently over the surface of the skin in the painful area for 10 to 20 seconds.
2. If touching this area causes pain or severe discomfort, stroke the area of skin around the painful area for 20 to 30 seconds. Try to remain relaxed and continue to breathe calmly. Work out how effective this is for you by doing an assessment. What effects do you get from stimulating the skin around the

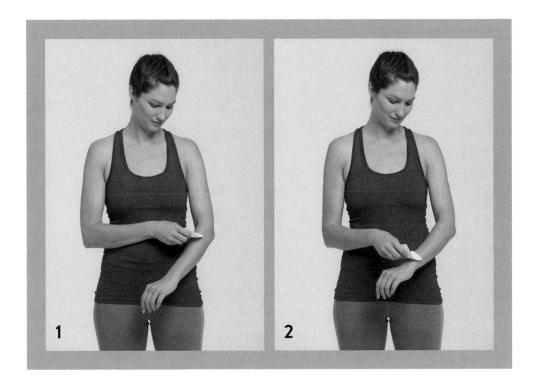

painful area? What effects do you get from stroking the painful area itself? If you don't get any negative effects from lightly touching one or both of these areas, then by all means include this stimulation in the following combinations.

❯ Stimulating the skin using vibration

Equipment: Z-Vibe

1. Do this exercise using the same method as for stimulating the skin using light touch, but instead of touching the skin with a cloth, test what happens if you apply gentle vibration using the Z-Vibe. Again, check the effect of this on the painful area.

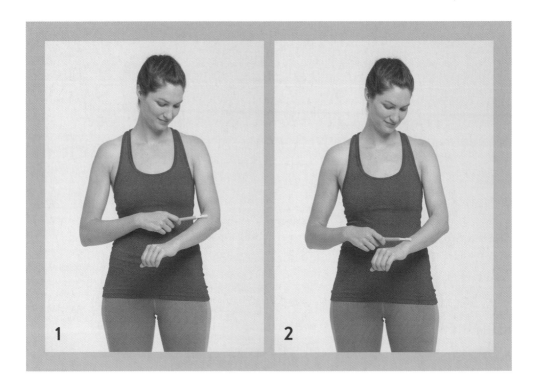

2. Now test the area of skin around the painful area. Make sure that you only apply the vibration to the very top layer of skin, using almost no pressure at all. Carry out each vibration for 20 to 30 seconds. Work out how effective this is for you by doing an assessment. What effects do you get from stimulating the skin around the painful area? What effects do you get from vibrating the painful area itself? If you don't get any negative effects from vibrating one or both of these areas, then by all means include this stimulation in the following combinations.

Categorising the variations of skin stimulation through light touch or vibration			
Exercise	Positive	Neutral/moderately positive	Save for later
Stimulating the skin using light touch (pages 284–285)			
Variation 1: Lightly touching the area of skin in the painful area			
Variation 2: Lightly touching the area of skin around the painful area			
Stimulating the skin using vibration (pages 285–286)			
Variation 1: Vibrating the area of skin in the painful area			
Variation 2: Vibrating the area of skin around the painful area			

Make a note of which of the four variations worked best for you and use this as part of your exercise combinations. This means performing the most effective variation while wearing an abdominal belt and doing tongue or breathing exercises. If you get a positive assessment result for more than one variation, alternate between them as part of your exercise combinations. If you find that none of the variations currently have positive effects or if they have negative effects, simply leave the skin stimulation exercise out for now and try testing it again in a few weeks.

We will now show you a variety of combinations that work well to gradually alleviate patterns of chronic pain. Feel free to warm up for these exercises by doing 20 to 30 seconds of olfactory perception (pages 92–93).

› Combination 6

Duration: 3 to 5 minutes

Equipment: Abdominal belt, heat pad, thin cloth or Z-Vibe

Exercise	Page
Wearing an abdominal belt	222
Variation: Applying the heat for longer	217
Stimulating the skin through light touch or vibration	284-286

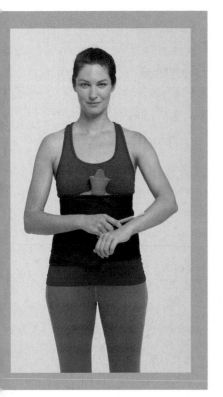

Preparation: Using the abdominal belt, tie a hot water bottle or heat pad to your stomach, pulling it tight to apply pressure. Make sure that the amount of pressure applied is comfortable for you. Pick up the cloth or Z-Vibe.

Stand or sit in a comfortable position. Lengthen your spine but keep it nice and relaxed. Allow your breath to flow smoothly and evenly. Start to gently stroke or vibrate the skin in or around the painful area using the stimulus that works best for you – either a cloth or the Z-Vibe. Continue to stimulate the area for 3 to 5 minutes. Make sure that you cover a large area of skin, and change the direction of your strokes from time to time. Try repeating this combination three to five times per day.

Note: You can vary the stimulus in this exercise by using a different cloth each time or using a different surface structure on the Z-Vibe. You can also make small but constant changes to the speed with which you stroke the skin. However, the most important thing is that you keep your breathing calm and relaxed and don't lose focus on how the skin feels.

› **Combination 7**   Duration: 3 to 5 minutes

Equipment: Abdominal belt, thin cloth or Z-Vibe

Exercise	Page
Wearing an abdominal belt	222
Stimulating the skin through light touch or vibration	284–286
'No-no' movements (horizontal)	66–67

Preparation: Wrap the abdominal belt tightly around your stomach, but not so tightly that the pressure is too uncomfortable. Pick up the cloth or Z-Vibe.

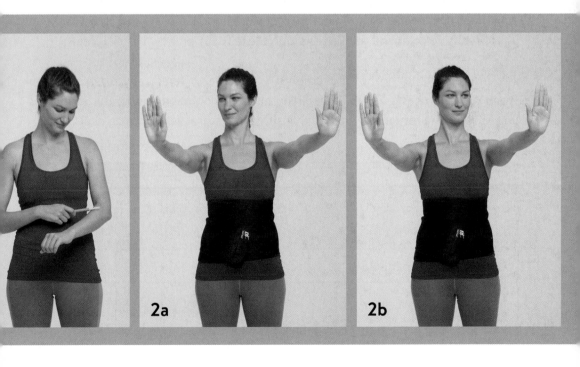

2a   2b

1. Stand or sit in a comfortable position. Lengthen your spine but keep it nice and relaxed. Allow your breath to flow smoothly and evenly. Start to gently stroke or vibrate the skin in or around the painful area using the stimulus that works best for you – either a cloth or the Z-Vibe. Continue to stimulate the area for 1 to 2 minutes. Make sure that you cover a large area of skin, and change the direction of your strokes from time to time.

2. **a+b** Then do 2 to 3 minutes of balance training by turning your head from side to side in a series of 'no-no' movements. Choose a speed that you find comfortable and that allows you to maintain control. You should try to do this combination of exercises three to five times per day.

Note: You're welcome to take a little break now and again to return to stroking the skin, before switching back to the head movements. Keep the skin stimulation varied by using a different cloth each time or using a different surface structure on the Z-Vibe. You can also make small but constant changes to the speed with which you stroke the skin. However, the most important thing is that you keep your breathing calm and relaxed and don't lose focus on how the skin feels.

Tip: Instead of the 'no-no' movements, you can also select any other exercise from the seven basic vestibular training exercises on pages 66 to 85, as long as you choose one for which you had a positive or neutral assessment result.

Categorising the combinations for chronic pain			
Combination	Positive	Neutral/moderately positive	Save for later
Combination 6 (page 288)			
Combination 7 (pages 289–290)			

Training recommendations for improving chronic pain

If you had positive assessment results for the previous combinations 6 and 7, then you should use them for at least 20 minutes a day, divided into four or five smaller sessions. You may also wish to incorporate whichever skin stimulation works best for you (cloth or Z-Vibe) into your daily routine for 4 to 6 minutes. If you haven't had positive assessment results for the combinations mentioned, despite adjusting the intensity, spend two to three weeks focusing on the respiratory training (pages 121–161), vestibular training (pages 66–85) and localising acoustic signals (pages 225–231) before coming back to the special combinations in this chapter.

Category 3: Emotional regulation

The best method for improving problems with emotional regulation – caused by interoceptive dysfunction – involves a combination of pressure on the abdomen, application of heat, and breathing exercises. As we saw in Chapter 1 from page 20 and in Chapter 7 from page 248, the cognitive, emotional and social aspects of our interoceptive awareness are regulated and governed by the anterior section of the insular cortex. You therefore need to improve the pattern of activation in the insular cortex from the back to the front, while also using certain exercises to target the anterior section of the insular cortex.

We recommend that you round off each combination by spending 3 to 5 minutes doing a body scan (pages 256–257) or mindfulness meditation focusing on breathing (pages 257–258). In the following section, we will show you two different combinations that bring together the most important aspects for this area.

> **Combination 8**   Duration: 8 to 15 minutes

Equipment: Abdominal belt, hot water bottle, Frolov respiratory training device or Relaxator

Exercise	Page
Wearing an abdominal belt	222
Variation: Applying the heat for longer	217
One of the variations of prolonged exhalation using the respiratory training devices: • Prolonged exhalation using the Relaxator • Prolonged exhalation using the Frolov respiratory training device	 148–149 150
Finish off with a body scan or mindfulness meditation	256–257 or 257–258

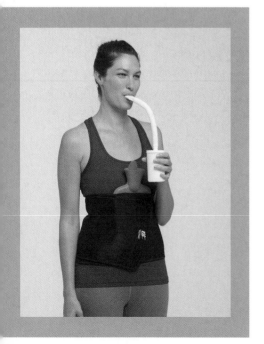

Preparation: Using the abdominal belt, tie a hot water bottle or heat pad to your stomach, applying light to moderate pressure. Make sure that the amount of pressure applied is comfortable for you.

Sit or stand in a comfortable position. Lengthen your spine but keep it nice and relaxed. Allow your breath to flow smoothly and evenly. Start with the Relaxator or the Frolov respiratory training device and use whichever variation of prolonged exhalation you find most comfortable and had a positive assessment result for. Breathe like this for between 5 and 10 minutes. Then finish off by spending 3 to 5 minutes doing a body scan or mindfulness meditation. Repeat this combination two or three times per day.

❯ **Combination 9**   **Duration: 8 to 15 minutes**

Equipment: Abdominal belt and Frolov respiratory training device or Relaxator

Exercise	Page
Wearing an abdominal belt	222
One of the variations of prolonged exhalation using the respiratory training devices: • Prolonged exhalation using the Relaxator • Prolonged exhalation using the Frolov respiratory training device	148–149 150
Finish off with a body scan or mindfulness meditation	256–257 or 257–258

Preparation: Fasten the abdominal belt tightly around your stomach, but not so tightly that the pressure is uncomfortable.

Sit or stand in a comfortable position. Lengthen your spine but keep it nice and relaxed. Allow your breath to flow smoothly and evenly. Start with the Relaxator or the Frolov respiratory training device and use whichever variation of prolonged exhalation you find most comfortable and had a positive assessment result for. Breathe like this for between 5 and 10 minutes. Then finish off by spending 3 to 5 minutes doing a body scan or mindfulness meditation. Repeat this combination two or three times per day.

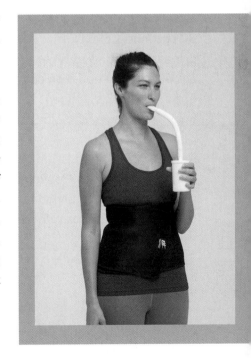

Categorising the combinations of exercises for improving emotional regulation			
Combination	Positive	Neutral/moderately positive	Save for later
Combination 8 (page 292)			
Combination 9 (page 293)			

Training recommendations for improving emotional regulation

If you want to see an improvement in your emotional regulation, you need to be doing at least 20 to 30 minutes of training per day. Combinations of pressure and heat, applied to the abdominal area, are particularly effective, especially when combined with one of the prolonged exhalation exercises described in combinations 8 and 9. You can also warm up for this training using the vagus nerve mobilisation exercises on pages 102–103 or the sensory stimulus of the auricular branch vagus nerve stimulation exercise on page 107. Brief stimulation for 20 to 30 seconds is plenty. If you feel that it is having a positive effect on you, you can pre-activate the vagus nerve using vibration for up to 2 minutes. Then carry out either Combination 8 on page 292 or Combination 9 on page 293, for which you got a positive assessment result, and finish off the training session with a short body scan (pages 256–257) or mindfulness meditation (pages 257–258).

Repeat the exercise two or three times a day, so that your overall training time is 20 to 30 minutes. You might want to supplement your training with exercises to activate the frontal lobe (pages 55–63), especially if you have difficulty controlling your impulses sufficiently.

Category 4: Digestive disorders

If you want to get a good handle on your digestive disorders and make lasting changes, you can combine all the exercises that activate the vagus nerve and parasympathetic system. As a basis for your training, it's always worth starting by applying pressure and heat to the stomach area, and combining this with one breathing exercise from Chapter 4 (page 123 onwards), one tongue or throat exercise for vagus nerve activation from Chapter 5 (page 186 onwards) or direct stimulation of the aural branches of the vagus nerve from Chapter 3 (pages 106–107). Use the exercises for which you had positive assessment results.

Because the vagus nerve sends anti-inflammatory signals to the organs, we would recommend that you also do the sensory stimulus of the auricular branch exercise for 2 or 3 minutes a day, as a standalone exercise to directly stimulate the vagus nerve. You should also try substituting this exercise regularly with other variations of vagus nerve stimulation. For example, you could combine the humming exercise with different breathing exercises. As a general rule, regulating digestive problems is a little like treating chronic pain or depressive moods, in that it takes a little longer to achieve noticeable effects. We therefore recommend that you invest 30 minutes a day in the training, and continue to practise for between four and six weeks.

❯ Combination 10   Duration: 3 to 5 minutes

Equipment: Abdominal belt, hot water bottle or heat pad

Exercise	Page
Wearing an abdominal belt	222
Variation: Applying the heat for longer	217
3D breathing	131
Tongue circles	191

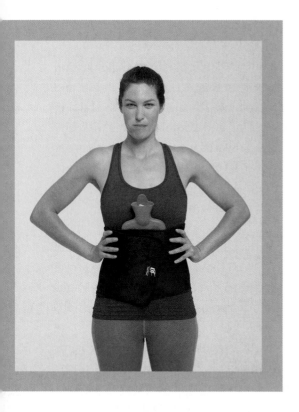

Preparation: Using the abdominal belt, tie a hot water bottle or heat pad to your stomach, pulling it tight to apply pressure. Make sure that the amount of pressure applied is comfortable for you.

Stand with your feet shoulder-distance apart. Lengthen your spine but keep it nice and relaxed. Allow your breath to flow smoothly and evenly. Now start your 3D breathing. Breathe softly and deeply in through your nose and slowly out through your nose. Once you have a feel for the rhythm of your breathing, start to circle your tongue as you breathe out. Continue this combination of exercises for 3 to 5 minutes at a time, and repeat three to five times throughout the day.

Note: Feel free to take a little break from tongue circles or switch to a different exercise such as tongue side to side (page 192). If you find it too difficult to combine tongue circles with the breathing exercise, you can also take a little break while you focus on tongue circles and then go back to the 3D breathing. Try to relax and find your own rhythm. Doing the exercise 'differentiating and identifying smells' (pages 92–93) for 20 to 30 seconds makes a really good warm-up for this exercise combination.

Tip: Rather than tongue circles you can use other tongue or throat exercises from Chapter 5 for which you had a positive assessment result, such as the tongue side to side (page 192), pushing the tongue out and pulling it in (page 193), humming (pages 204–205) or – if you have made good progress – positioning the tongue correctly (pages 190–191) or active tongue stretch (pages 196–197).

❯ **Combination 11** Duration: 3 to 5 minutes

Equipment: Abdominal belt, hot water bottle or heat pad, Relaxator, Z-Vibe

Exercise	Page
Wearing an abdominal belt	222
Variation: Applying the heat for longer	217
Prolonged exhalation using the Relaxator	148–149
Sensory stimulus of the auricular branch	107

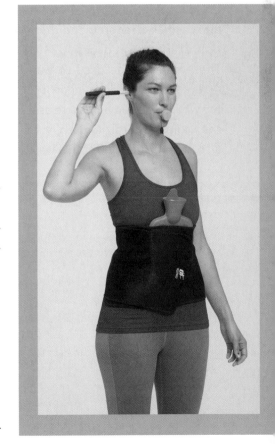

Preparation: Using the abdominal belt, tie a hot water bottle or heat pad to your stomach, pulling it tight to apply pressure. Make sure that the amount of pressure applied is comfortable for you. Pick up the Relaxator.

Stand or sit in a comfortable position. Lengthen your spine but keep it nice and relaxed. Allow your breath to flow smoothly and evenly. Place the Relaxator loosely between your lips and begin to carry out prolonged exhalations through the device. Take three or four calm breaths. Then start the vibration in your right ear. If you find vibrating the ear uncomfortable, feel free to take a short break and then start again. Continue this combination of exercises for 3 to 5 minutes at a time, and repeat three to five times throughout the day.

Tip: Rather than prolonged exhalation using the Relaxator, you can use the Frolov respiratory training device instead (page 150), or any other prolonged exhalation technique.

Categorising the combinations for improving digestive disorders			
Combination	Positive	Neutral/moderately positive	Save for later
Combination 10 (pages 295–296)			
Combination 11 (page 297)			

Training recommendations for improving digestive disorders

Digestion is a complex internal process. It takes time to achieve changes in this area. For sustainable and lasting improvement of digestive problems, you need to train for at least 20 to 30 minutes per day. In addition to the combinations given here, we also recommend that you regularly perform the vagus nerve mobilisation exercises on pages 102–103 and the diaphragm stretch on pages 123–124. These can also be used to warm up for training using combinations 10 and 11. Alternatively, you can incorporate any of the vestibular exercises (pages 66–85) for which you had a positive assessment result. Doing prolonged exhalation using the Frolov respiratory training device (page 149) for at least 20 minutes per day is also an extremely effective way of treating digestive problems.

Category 5: Pelvic floor dysfunction

As you already know from Chapter 4 'Breathing and the pelvic floor', the pelvic floor is closely connected to your breathing and responds well to tongue exercises. So, this isn't primarily about improving the activity pattern of the insular cortex. These two aspects should therefore always be included in the exercise combinations or used as an additional warm-up exercise. One of the most important aspects of successful pelvic floor training is activating the neural pathways. Just exercising the pelvic floor muscles in isolation often won't get you where you want to be, especially if you've been experiencing your symptoms for a long time. The most effective way to warm up for your training is to carry out exercises that activate the supplementary motor areas of the brain (page 110). The following combination is probably the most effective way of preparing your nervous system for pelvic floor training.

> ## › Combination 12 for pre-activating the pelvic floor
Duration: 20 to 30 seconds

Equipment: Z-Vibe

Exercise	Page
Vibrating the front teeth	110
Alternating between opening and closing the hands	111

Tip: Instead of alternating between opening and closing your hands, you can also do bilateral wrist rotations and the two corresponding variations on pages 112 to 114.

a+b: Stand with your feet hip-width apart. Lengthen your spine but keep it nice and relaxed. Allow your breath to flow smoothly and evenly. Turn on the Z-Vibe and place it loosely between your incisors. Begin to alternate between opening and closing your hands. Continue this stimulation for 20 to 30 seconds.

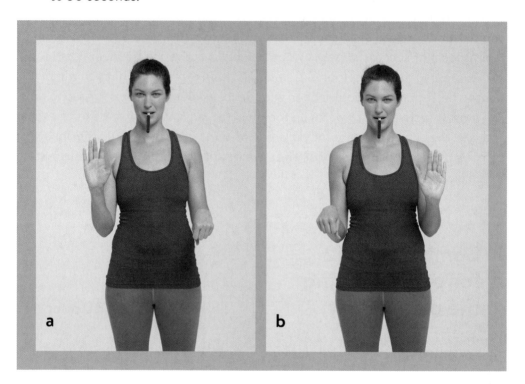

Training recommendations for pelvic floor dysfunction

To see long-term improvements, especially in pelvic floor problems that have been bothering you for a long time, you need to be doing two 10 to 15-minute training sessions per day. Make sure you always do a thorough warm-up session first. For this, you can start your training with any of the tongue exercises from pages 188 to 199 for which you had positive assessment results. Then move on to either 2 to 3 minutes of prolonged exhalation (pages 146–149) or the 3D breathing exercise or one of its variations on pages 131 to 140. Make sure you pick one for which you had a positive assessment result. For the final stage of the warm-up, use Combination 12 with a hand movement that you are able to coordinate well. Finish with one to three exercises of your choice from the pelvic floor exercises on pages 170 to 177.

About the authors

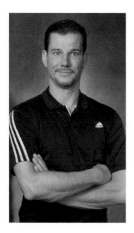

Lars Lienhard, sports scientist and former performance athlete, works as a trainer and consultant in high-performance sport. He has been training world-class athletes in a range of sporting disciplines for many years. He was one of the specialists responsible for taking care of the German national football team during the 2014 World Cup in Brazil. In 2016, he accompanied the German athletes to the summer Olympic games in Rio de Janeiro. Lienhard has been applying his neurocentric approach – based on the work of Dr Eric Cobb – to athletics training since 2010. He regularly holds workshops, seminars and talks, sharing his experience in the field with trainers, athletes, sporting federations and clubs.

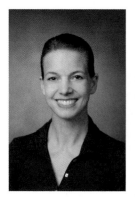

Ulla Schmid-Fetzer, author and former dance performance athlete, completed the Z-Health training course to become a neuroathletics trainer in record time and is now one of the few fully certified trainers in the whole of Europe. As a trainer in the field of competitive dance, she trains a wide range of athletes at all stages in their careers – from up-and-coming talents to world champions. As well as working as a trainer and adviser in the field of neuroathletics, she is also involved with the rehabilitation of professional national league footballers, and has recently begun pursuing the field of neurocentric health optimisation. Ulla Schmid-Fetzer is the author of the world's first book on neurocentric training.

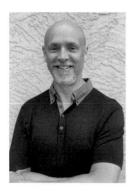

Dr Eric Cobb, founder of Z-Health® Performance Solutions, is one of the world's leading experts in innovative, neurologically-focused rehabilitation and sports performance programmes. Dr Cobb's passion for people's fitness and for developing practical ways to implement complex training content is evident in the fun and enjoyable courses and professional certifications offered by his team worldwide. With over 3000 certified Z-Health trainers across the globe, Dr Cobb's goal is to establish neurocentric training and therapy in hospitals, gyms and sports centres all over the world.

Equipment

For sight and touch exercises

We use a wide range of tools and equipment in this book. Some of these are available to buy online from Perform Better Europe. They sell a 'Neuro Athletic Starter Set', which contains the training cards used in this book (near/far cards and saccade cards) as well as the VisionStick. The Z-Vibe and other equipment can also be purchased individually.

https://www.perform-better.de/en/shop/others/neuro-athletics-equipment/

For breathing exercises

The Relaxator, the Expand-A-Lung and the Frolov respiratory training device are available to order online, for example from **www.amazon.co.uk or www.amazon. com**.

For vestibular and hearing exercises

In Chapter 8, we use bone conduction headphones. Unlike normal headphones, these are not placed over the ears, but rather directly onto the temporal bones above the ears. The frequencies are conducted into the ear through the bones. The headphones come in two versions. They can be connected to your mobile device via Bluetooth or using a cable. To select the desired frequencies, you will also need a frequency generator (see 'Apps' on page 304). The headphones are available online from various suppliers and there are several different models available. The prices differ considerably. Watch out for the quality and the manufacturer's specifications, and remember it's always worth reading user ratings and reviews.

We recommend the bone conduction headphones made by the American company Sound for Life. They developed Forbrain® and Soundsory®. Both systems use bone conduction. However, the headphones with the Forbrain® system are placed onto the temporal bones, whereas the Soundsory® headphones completely cover your outer ears and therefore also transmit airborne sound. In the US, both systems can be purchased directly from **www.forbrain.com** and **soundsory.com**. In the UK, the products are available from **www.amazon.co.uk**.

Apps

In Chapter 7, we recommend using the *Headspace* app for mindfulness training. This is available from the app store on your mobile device.

To use the bone conduction headphones, you also need a frequency generator in order to adjust the frequencies for the exercises in Chapter 8. The apps *Function Generator Pro* and *Tone Pacer* work really well.

In Chapter 3, we recommend a few different apps and games for training the frontal lobe and improving impulse control. These are *Stroop Test*, *Dual N-Back* and *Go/no-go*. In the app store, you will find even more games that you can use. Some of the games are also available online or can be downloaded onto your tablet.

Want to know more?

On the following pages, we have put together a list of interesting and relevant studies, journals and websites where you can find out more about the scientific principles behind this incredible phenomenon; this is the first time that this subject has been covered so comprehensively in a book designed for a general audience. We would also like to recommend a few books, some originally published in German and some in English, which explore individual topics we've touched upon, such as interoception or the insular cortex. The majority of the existing literature on these topics is written in English.

Recommended studies and websites

Blog by Neuroskeptic: *Does the Motor Cortex Inhibit Movement?* In: Discover – Science for the Curious (3 November 2016), http://blogs.discovermagazine.com/neuroskeptic/2016/11/03/motor-cortex-inhibit/

Cechetto, D. F.: *Cortical Control of the Autonomic Nervous System.* In: Experimental Physiology, 99 (2), pp. 326–331 (18 October 2013), https://doi.org/10.1113/expphysiol.2013.075192

Ceunen, Erik; Vlaeyen, Johan W. S; Van Diest, Ilse: *On the Origin of Interoception*. In: Frontiers in Psychology 7 (23 May 2016), https://doi.org/10.3389/fpsyg.2016.00743

Deen, B.; Pitskel, N. B.; Pelphrey, K. A. (2010): *Three Systems of Insular Functional Connectivity Identified with Cluster Analysis*. In: Cerebral Cortex, 21 (7), pp. 1498–1506, https://doi.org/10.1093/cercor/bhq186

Gilbert, J. W.; Vogt, M.; Windsor, R. E.; Mick, G. E.; Richardson, G. B.; Storey, B. B.; Herder, S. L.; Ledford, S.; Abrams, D. A.; Theobald, M. K. (2014): *Vestibular Dysfunction in Patients With Chronic Pain or Underlying Neurologic Disorders*. In: The Journal of the American Osteopathic Association, 114 (3), pp. 172–178, https://doi.org/10.7556/jaoa.2014.034

Gogolla, N. (2017): *The Insular Cortex*. In: Current Biology, 27 (12), pp. R580–R586, https://doi.org/10.1016/j.cub.2017.05.010

Gotink, R. A.; Meijboom, R.; Vernooij, M. W.; Smits, M.; Hunink, M. G. (2016): *8-Week Mindfulness Based Stress Reduction Induces Brain Changes Similar to Traditional Long-Term Meditation Practice – A Systematic Review*. In: Brain and Cognition, 108, pp. 32–41

Haase, Lori; Stewart, Jennifer L.; Youssef, Brittany; May, April C.; Isakovic, Sara; Simmons, Alan N.; Johnson, Douglas C.; Potterat, Eric G.; Paulus, Martin P.: *When the Brain Does Not Adequately Feel the Body: Links Between Low Resilience and Interoception*. In: Biological Psychology 113 (January 2016), pp. 37–45, https://doi.org/10.1016/j.biopsycho.2015.11.004

Jené, K. (2012): *MBSR für Patienten mit chronischen Schmerzen* [MBSR for patients with chronic pain]. In: Angewandte Schmerztherapie und Palliativmedizin [Applied pain management and palliative medicine], 5 (3), pp. 46 et seq.

Kim, S.; Lee, D. (2011): *Prefrontal Cortex and Impulsive Decision Making*. In: Biological Psychiatry, 69 (12), pp. 1140–1146 (21 August 2010), https://doi.org/10.1016/j.biopsych.2010.07.005

Levinson, A. J.; Fitzgerald, P. B.; Favalli, G.; Blumberger, D. M.; Daigle, M.; Daskalakis, Z. J. (2010): *Evidence of Cortical Inhibitory Deficits in Major Depressive Disorder.* In: Biological Psychiatry, 67 (5), pp. 458–464, https://doi.org/10.1016/j.biopsych.2009.09.025

Paulus, Martin P.; Stein, Murray B.: *Interoception in Anxiety and Depression.* In: Brain Structure and Function 214 (5–6), (June 2010), pp. 451–463, https://doi.org/10.1007/s00429-010-0258-9

Pavuluri, Mani; May, Amber and 1 Pediatric Mood Disorders Program and Pediatric Brain Research and Intervention Center, Department of Psychiatry, College of Medicine, University of Illinois at Chicago, Chicago, IL 60608, USA (2015): *I Feel, Therefore, I Am: The Insula and Its Role in Human Emotion, Cognition and the Sensory-Motor System.* In: AIMS Neuroscience 2 (1), pp. 18–27, https://doi.org/10.3934/Neuroscience.2015.1.18

Radley, J. J. (2012): Toward a Limbic Cortical Inhibitory Network: *Implications for Hypothalamic-Pituitary-Adrenal Responses Following Chronic Stress.* In: Frontiers in Behavioral Neuroscience, 6, 7, https://doi.org/10.3389/fnbeh.2012.00007

Russo, Scott J.; Murrough, James W.; Han, Ming-Hu; Charney, Dennis S.; Nestler, Eric J.: *Neurobiology of Resilience.* In: Nature Neuroscience 15 (11), pp. 1475–1484 (November 2012), https://doi.org/10.1038/nn.3234

Seth, Anil K.: *Interoceptive Inference, Emotion, and the Embodied Self.* In: Trends in Cognitive Sciences 17 (11), pp. 565–573 (November 2013), https://doi.org/10.1016/j.tics.2013.09.007

Shelley, B. P.; Trimble, M. R. (2004): *The Insular Lobe of Reil – Its Anatamico-Functional, Behavioural and Neuropsychiatric Attributes in Humans – A Review.* In: The World Journal of Biological Psychiatry, 5 (4), pp. 176–200, https://doi.org/10.1080/15622970410029933

Silva, D. R. D.; Osório, R. A. L.; Fernandes, A. B. (2018): *Influence of Neural Mobilization in the Sympathetic Slump Position on the Behavior of the Autonomic Nervous*

System. In: Research on Biomedical Engineering, 34 (4), pp. 329–336, http://dx. doi.org/10.1590/2446-4740.180037

Starr, C. J.; Sawaki, L.; Wittenberg, G. F.; Burdette, J. H.; Oshiro, Y.; Quevedo, A. S.; Coghill, R. C. (2009): *Roles of the Insular Cortex in the Modulation of Pain: Insights from Brain Lesions*. In: Journal of Neuroscience, 29 (9), pp. 2684–2694, https://doi.org/10.1523/JNEUROSCI.5173-08.2009

Uddin, Lucina Q.; Nomi, Jason S.; Hébert-Seropian, Benjamin; Ghaziri, Jimmy; Boucher, Olivier: *Structure and Function of the Human Insula*. In: Journal of Clinical Neurophysiology: Official Publication of the American Electroencephalographic Society 34 (4), pp. 300–306 (July 2017), https://doi.org/10.1097/WNP.0000000000000377

Zaccaro, Andrea; Piarulli, Andrea; Laurino, Marco; Garbella, Erika; Menicucci, Danilo; Neri, Bruno; Gemignani, Angelo: *How Breath-Control Can Change Your Life: A Systematic Review on Psycho-Physiological Correlates of Slow Breathing*. In: Frontiers in Human Neuroscience 12, p. 353 (17 September 2018), https://doi.org/10.3389/fnhum.2018.00353

https://scholar.google.co.uk
Google Scholar is the world's largest academic search engine. It is owned by Google LLC and allows users to carry out general literature searches for scientific documents. Here you will find articles from the internet, some of which are free and some of which required paid access. If you wish to read up on this topic in more depth, we recommend entering search terms such as 'insular cortex', 'interoceptive awareness' or 'resilience'.

Recommendations for further reading

Books published in German

Berndt, Christina (2015): *Resilienz. Das Geheimnis der psychischen Widerstandskraft. Was uns stark macht gegen Stress, Depressionen und Burn-out*. (Resilience: The Secret of Harnessing Your Inner Resources). 7th edition, dtv, Munich

Doidge, Norman (2017): *Neustart im Kopf. Wie sich unser Gehirn selbst repariert. [The Brain That Changes Itself]*. 3rd edition, Campus Verlag, Frankfurt am Main

Jacobson, Edmund (2017): *Entspannung als Therapie: Progressive Relaxation in Theorie und Praxis (Leben lernen). [Progressive Relaxation]*. 8th edition, Klett-Cotta, Stuttgart

Jost, Wolfgang H. (2009): *Neurokoloproktologie – Neurologie des Beckenbodens. (Neurology of the Pelvic Floor)*. 2nd edition, Uni-Med, Bremen

Kabat-Zinn, Jon (2013): *Gesund durch Meditation. Das große Buch der Selbstheilung mit MBSR. [Full Catastrophe Living: How to Cope With Stress, Pain and Illness Using Mindfulness Meditation]*. Knaur Taschenbuch Verlag, Munich

Kabat-Zinn, Jon (2015): *Im Alltag Ruhe finden. [Falling Awake: How to Practise Mindfulness in Everyday Life]*. 6th edition, Knaur Taschenbuch Verlag, Munich

Kipp, Markus; Radlanski, Kalinka (2017): *Neuroanatomie: nachschlagen, lernen, verstehen. (Neuroanatomy: Researching, Learning, Understanding)*. KVM – Der Medizinverlag, Berlin

Lienhard, Lars (2019): *Training beginnt im Gehirn. Mit Neuroathletik die sportliche Leistung verbessern. (Training Begins in the Brain: Improving Athletic Performance With Neuroathletics)*. riva Verlag, Munich

Rosenberg, Stanley (2018): *Der Selbstheilungsnerv. So bringt der Vagus-Nerv Psyche und Körper ins Gleichgewicht. [Activating the Healing Power of the Vagus Nerve]*. VAK Verlag, Kirchzarten

Schmid-Fetzer, Ulla (2018): *Neuroathletiktraining. Grundlagen und Praxis des neurozentrierten Trainings. (Neuroathletics Training: The Theory and Practice of Neurocentric Training)*. Pflaum Verlag, Munich

Schnack, Prof. Gerd (2016): *Der große Ruhe-Nerv. Soforthilfen gegen Stress und Burn-out. (The Great Calmness Nerve: Instant Alleviation of Stress and Burn-Out).* Verlag Herder, Freiburg

Trepel, Martin (2015): *Neuroanatomie: Struktur und Funktion. (Neuroanatomy: Structure and Function).* 6th edition, Urban & Fischer Verlag, Munich and Jena

Books published in English

Beck, Randy. W. (2007): *Functional Neurology for Practitioners of Manual Medicine.* Churchill Livingstone, London

Benedetto, Fabrizio (2011): *The Patient's Brain: The Neuroscience Behind the Doctor-Patient Relationship.* Oxford University Press, Oxford

Calais-Germain, Blandine (2006): *Anatomy of Breathing.* Eastland Press, Seattle

Calais-Germain, Blandine (1996): *Anatomy of Movement: Exercises.* Eastland Press, Seattle

Carr, Janet H.; Shepherd, Roberta B. (2010): *Neurological Rehabilitation: Optimizing Motor Performance.* Churchill Livingstone, London

Craig, A. D. (2015): *How Do You Feel? An Interoceptive Moment With Your Neurobiological Self.* Princeton University Press, New Jersey

Gutman, Sharon A. (2016): *Quick Reference Neuroscience for Rehabilitation Professionals: The Essential Neurologic Principles Underlying Rehabilitation Practice.* 3rd edition, Slack Incorporated, Thorofare

Hatch, Dr John D. (2017): *The Basis of Brain Rehab.* CreateSpace Independent Publishing Platform

Herdman, Susan J.; Clendaniel, Richard A. (2014): *Vestibular Rehabilitation.* 4th edition, F. A. Davis Company, Philadelphia

Kandel, Eric R.; Schwartz, James H.; Jessell, Thomas M.; Siegelbaum, Steven A.; Hudspeth, A. J. (2013): *Principles of Neural Science*. 5th edition, McGraw-Hill Education, New York

Lundy-Ekman, Laurie (2018): *Neuroscience: Fundamentals for Rehabilitation*. 5th edition, Elsevier, Oxford

Mahler, Kelly (2017): *Interoception: The Eighth Sensory System: Practical Solutions for Improving Self-Regulation, Self-Awareness and Social Understanding*. AAPC Publishing, Lenexa

Melzack, Ronald; Katz, Joel (2006): *Pain in the 21st Century: The Neuromatrix and Beyond*. In: Young, Gerald; Kane, Andrew W.; Nicholson, Keith: Psychological Knowledge in Court: PTSD, Pain, and TBI. Springer Science, New York, pp. 129–148

Moseley, G. Lorimer; Butler, David S. (2017): *Explain Pain Supercharged*. NOI Group Publications, Adelaide

Myers, Thomas W. (2014): *Anatomy Trains: Myofascial Meridians for Manual and Movement Therapists*. 3rd edition, Churchill Livingstone, London

Porges, Stephen W. (2017): *The Pocket Guide to the Polyvagal Theory: The Transformative Power of Feeling Safe*. W. W. Norton & Company, New York

Tsakiris, Manos; De Preester, Helena (2019): *The Interoceptive Mind: From Homeostasis to Awareness*. Oxford University Press, Oxford

Wilson-Pauwels, Linda; Akesson, Elizabeth J.; Spacey, Siân D.; Stewart, Patricia A. (2010): *Cranial Nerves: Function and Dysfunction*. 3rd edition, PMPH-USA, Cary

Scientific studies and articles

Clark, Andy (2013). *Whatever Next? Predictive Brains, Situated Agents, and the Future of Cognitive Science*. In: Behavioral and Brain Sciences, 36 (3), pp. 181–204

Downing, Keith L. (2009). *Predictive Models in the Brain*. In: Connection Science, 21 (1), pp. 39–74

Gaerlan, Mary Grace (2010). *The Role of Visual, Vestibular, and Somatosensory Systems in Postural Balance*. (Doctoral thesis), University of Nevada, Las Vegas

Kleim, Jeffrey A.; Jones, Theresa A. (2008). *Principles of Experience-Dependent Neural Plasticity: Implications for Rehabilitation After Brain Damage*. In: Journal of Speech, Language, and Hearing Research, 51 (1), pp. 225–239

Wildenberg, Joe C.; Tyler, Mitchell E.; Danilov, Yuri P.; Kaczmarek, Kurt A.; Meyerand, Mary E. (2013): *Altered Connectivity of the Balance Processing Network After Tongue Stimulation in Balance-Impaired Individuals*. In: Brain Connectivity, 3 (1), pp. 87–97

List of exercises

Chapter 2: Assessments – quick tests for lasting success

Chapter 3: Laying the foundations for optimal vagus nerve training

Chapter 4: Breathing and the pelvic floor

Chapter 5: Tongue and throat

Chapter 6: Touch, sound and vision for interoceptive awareness

Chapter 7: Body awareness and mindfulness

Chapter 8: Specific training plans to improve your health issues

Index